AF614681

New Insights on Cerebrospinal Fluid

Edited by Pinar Kuru Bektasoglu

Published in London, United Kingdom

New Insights on Cerebrospinal Fluid
http://dx.doi.org/10.5772/intechopen.1000434
Edited by Pinar Kuru Bektasoglu

Contributors
Babu Paturi, Gurjit Nagra, Kanwal Altaf Malik, Lauren Harbaugh, Li Zhang, Mariana-Alis Neagoe, Pinar Kuru Bektasoglu, Sarah Arianna Mirkhaef, Stephane Maingard

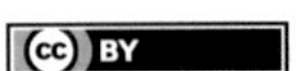

First published in London, United Kingdom, 2024 by IntechOpen
IntechOpen is the global imprint of INTECHOPEN LIMITED, registered in England and Wales, registration number: 11086078, 167-169 Great Portland Street, London, W1W 5PF, United Kingdom

British Library Cataloguing-in-Publication Data
A catalogue record for this book is available from the British Library

Additional hard and PDF copies can be obtained from orders@intechopen.com

New Insights on Cerebrospinal Fluid
Edited by Pinar Kuru Bektasoglu
p. cm.
Print ISBN 978-0-85466-506-8
Online ISBN 978-0-85466-505-1
eBook (PDF) ISBN 978-0-85466-507-5

For EU product safety concerns:
IN TECH d.o.o., Prolaz Marije Krucifikse Kozulić 3, 51000 Rijeka, Croatia,
info@intechopen.com or visit our website at intechopen.com.

Meet the editor

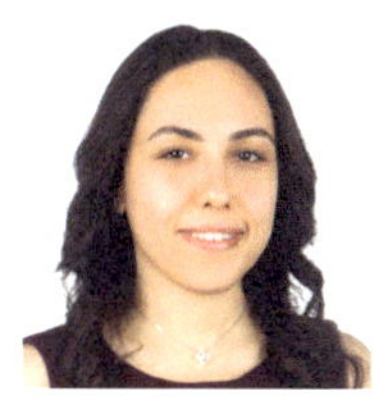

Dr. Pinar Kuru Bektaşoğlu is working as a neurosurgery consultant at Istanbul Fatih Sultan Mehmet Education and Research Hospital. She graduated from Marmara University School of Medicine, Turkey, in 2014. She completed her neurosurgical residency in 2021 and her Ph.D. in physiology at Marmara University Institute of Health Sciences, also in 2021. She worked as a research fellow in the Department of Neurological Surgery at Yeditepe University, Turkiye, for six months studying white matter fiber dissection. She has given more than 80 presentations at international and national meetings and published 50 papers in peer-reviewed journals. She also edited four books and wrote 11 book chapters. She has a keen interest in neurovascular and neuro-oncological surgeries and translational neuroscience.

Contents

Preface

Cerebrospinal fluid is an essential ultrafiltrate of plasma within brain ventricles and subarachnoid space. In this book project, we focus on the diagnostic role of cerebrospinal fluid and its future potential. Recent advances in molecular biology techniques widened the use of cerebrospinal fluid as a diagnostic and prognostic tool. You will find answers in this book for when to apply for cerebrospinal fluid analysis and what the current role of cerebrospinal fluid analysis is in infectious diseases, brain trauma, neuroinflammation, and neurodegenerative diseases. Also, we will discuss hydrocephalus and current treatment strategies. I hope you will find answers to your related questions and that we may give some inspiration for your future projects.

Pinar Kuru Bektasoglu, MD, Ph.D.
Istanbul Fatih Sultan Mehmet Education and Research Hospital,
Department of Neurosurgery,
Istanbul, Türkiye

Chapter 1

Introductory Chapter: New Insights on Cerebrospinal Fluid

Pinar Kuru Bektasoglu

1. Introduction

Cerebrospinal fluid (CSF) is an essential liquid circulating around the central nervous system (CNS). Besides its main physiological role, it also serves as a diagnostic tool. Some CNS infections are already diagnosed and followed by CSF analysis. Recent advances in molecular biology technology help detecting small amounts of proteins or nucleic acids and the diagnostic spectrum widens rapidly for CSF. In traumatic brain injury (TBI), some structural protein levels such as tau, glial fibrillary acidic protein (GFAP), neurofilament light (NF-L) polypeptide, and intracellular soluble molecules such as S100-B, UCH-L1 can indicate the brain injury [1]. As liquid biopsy biomarkers, circulating tumor cells (CTCs) or DNAs in CSF could give clue about CNS malignancies [2]. Increased IgG oligoclonal bands (OCBs) are important in the diagnosis and follow-up of multiple sclerosis (MS) [3]. The ratio of two amyloid β (Aβ) proteins ($A\beta_{42/40}$) is associated with the progression of Alzheimer's disease (AD) [4]. In this introductory chapter, I will briefly focus on recent advances in the diagnostic spectrum of CSF examination in neurotrauma, neuro-oncology, neuroinflammation, and neurodegeneration.

2. Current updates

2.1 Neurotrauma

Rather than being one disease, mild, moderate, and severe TBI are distinct pathobiological outcomes brought on by diverse types and intensities of mechanical forces [1]. The most widely used "neural damage markers" nowadays are those released by stressed, wounded, and dying neurons and astroglia, which include intracellular soluble molecules like UCH-L1, neuron-specific enolase (NSE), and S100B; structural proteins like GFAP, NF-L, and tau.

Elevated UCH-L1/GFAP levels almost invariably correspond with a positive CT scan, but not the other way around since elevated UCH-L1/GFAP levels may or may not imply structural damage that can be seen by imaging. UCH-L1 was discovered to be higher 1 hour after damage in a pilot investigation of patients with mild to moderate TBI. It was also found to be linked with injury severity, the Glasgow Coma Scale (GCS) score, and positive lesion findings on CT imaging.

Tau proteins, NF-L peptides, and phosphorylated neurofilament heavy peptides are examples of fluid indicators of acute axonal damage. NF-L are expressed in

IntechOpen

large-caliber myelinated axons in the spinal cord and deeper brain layers, whereas tau proteins are naturally present in thin, nonmyelinated axons of cortical interneurons. Total tau protein levels are increased in ventricular CSF in cases of severe TBI. These levels are correlated with the size, severity, and prognosis of the lesion [5].

2.2 Neuro-oncology

In neuro-oncology, clinical care has changed to an integrated approach that integrates imaging and histopathology data with molecular profiles. Using a non-invasive technique called liquid biopsy, one can identify particular tumor biomarkers that circulate in bodily fluids such as CSF, and therefore capture the molecular diversity of the entire tumor. However, the application of liquid biopsy in clinical settings has been limited due to the low presence and short half-life of tumor-derived biomarkers, particularly in malignancies of the CNS [2]. Tumor-specific mRNA, microRNAs (miRNA), proteins, extracellular vesicles (EV), circulating tumor DNA (ctDNA), CTCs, and the recently identified tumor-educated platelets (TEP) are a few examples of these tumoral components. With the potential to greatly advance both the diagnostic and therapeutic aspects of brain tumor liquid biopsies, targeted ultrasound-enhanced disruption of the blood–brain barrier heralds a new era in the field. The most recent and comprehensive systematic review of CSF as a biomarker in neuro-oncology was published by Mikolajewicz et al. [6].

2.3 Neuroinflammation and neurodegeneration

The gold standard for MS diagnosis, according to the most recent revision of McDonald's criteria, has been an OCB determination in the CSF. But as of late, the determination of the kappa free light chain (κFLC) index has become more and more relevant, offering a quick, easy, and dependable way to save money and time. Furthermore, similar to OCB detection, the κFLC index exhibits good specificity, although sensitivity varies because of various cut-off values. As things stand, one of the biggest obstacles to this biomarker's use in clinical settings is the absence of a defined cut-off value that would enable patients with MS to be distinguished from healthy individuals as well as those with other neurodegenerative illnesses [7].

Alzheimer's disease is the most common form of age-associated dementia. Early diagnosis of this neurodegenerative disease could help with early intervention and slow the progression of the disease process. It is well known that biomarkers helpful for the diagnosis of AD include decreases in CSF concentrations of tau species, which are markers of axonal damage and neurofibrillary tangles, and increases in $A\beta_{42}$, a sign of amyloidosis [4]. Crucially, research on these CSF biochemical indicators for AD has demonstrated that it is possible to predict the transition from mild cognitive impairment to AD dementia with >80% accuracy. A comprehensive literature stated that in order to increase the proportion of patients with an accurate diagnosis, the CSF Aβ42/40 ratio should be utilized when analyzing CSF AD biomarkers, as opposed to the absolute amount of CSF Aβ42.

Parkinson' disease (PD) exhibits great diversity among patients [8]. The PD-specific characteristics were linked to tau, Aβ42, and α-Synuclein in addition to PD, indicating that the three proteins work in concert to contribute to structural alterations in PD.

DOI: http://dx.doi.org/10.5772/intechopen.1007032

3. Conclusion and future insights

The clinical importance of the diagnostic and prognostic role of CSF is expanding with the improved techniques for liquid biopsy. It can be foreseen that combining the CSF biomarker data with other well-established, frequently used clinical diagnostic tools through the use of machine learning skills and artificial intelligence approaches will give the doctor useful information to diagnose and follow-up the patients with various neurological disorders.

Author details

Pinar Kuru Bektasoglu
Department of Neurosurgery, Istanbul Fatih Sultan Mehmet Education and Research Hospital, Istanbul, Türkiye

*Address all correspondence to: drpinarkuru@gmail.com

References

[1] Agoston DV, Helmy A. Fluid-based protein biomarkers in traumatic brain injury: The view from the bedside. International Journal of Molecular Sciences. 2023;**24**(22):16267. DOI: 10.3390/ijms242216267

[2] Khalili N, Shooli H, Hosseini N, Fathi Kazerooni A, Familiar A, Bagheri S, et al. Adding value to liquid biopsy for brain tumors: The role of imaging. Cancers (Basel). 2023;**15**(21):5198. DOI: 10.3390/cancers15215198

[3] Tunç A, Seferoğlu M, Sıvacı AÖ, Köktürk MD, Akbaş AA, Bozkurt B, et al. Oligoclonal band count as a marker of disease activity and progression in multiple sclerosis: A multicenter study. Journal of Clinical Neuroscience. 2024;**126**:353-360. DOI: 10.1016/j.jocn.2024.07.013

[4] Hansson O, Lehmann S, Otto M, Zetterberg H, Lewczuk P. Advantages and disadvantages of the use of the CSF amyloid β (Aβ) 42/40 ratio in the diagnosis of Alzheimer's disease. Alzheimer's Research & Therapy. 2019;**11**(1):34. DOI: 10.1186/s13195-019-0485-0

[5] Zhang J, Puvenna V, Janigro D. Biomarkers of traumatic brain injury and their relationship to pathology. In: Laskowitz D, Grant G, editors. Translational Research in Traumatic Brain Injury. Boca Raton (FL): CRC Press/Taylor and Francis Group; 2016. Chapter 12. Available from: https://www.ncbi.nlm.nih.gov/books/NBK326724/#

[6] Mikolajewicz N, Yee PP, Bhanja D, Trifoi M, Miller AM, Metellus P, et al. Systematic review of cerebrospinal fluid biomarker discovery in neuro-oncology: A roadmap to standardization and clinical application. Journal of Clinical Oncology. 2024;**42**(16):1961-1974. DOI: 10.1200/JCO.23.01621

[7] Maglio G, D'Agostino M, Caronte FP, Pezone L, Casamassimi A, Rienzo M, et al. Multiple sclerosis: From the application of oligoclonal bands to novel potential biomarkers. International Journal of Molecular Sciences. 2024;**25**(10):5412. DOI: 10.3390/ijms25105412

[8] Zheng L, Zhou C, Mao C, Xie C, You J, Cheng W, et al. Contrastive machine learning reveals Parkinson's disease specific features associated with disease severity and progression. Communications Biology. 2024;7(1):954. DOI: 10.1038/s42003-024-06648-x

Chapter 2

Hydrocephalus: A Review of Etiology Driven Treatment Strategies

Sarah Arianna Mirkhaef, Lauren Harbaugh and Gurjit Nagra

Abstract

Hydrocephalus is a broad term usually understood as cerebrospinal fluid (CSF) accumulation resulting in cerebral ventricular system expansion. The production of CSF is by the choroid plexus in lateral ventricles, flowing between the third and fourth ventricles and eventually to the subarachnoid space. It is critical for proper neuronal function. Hydrocephalus is a neurological pathology linked to high morbidity from neurocognitive and motor impairment. It is classified as either communicating or non-communicating. Communicating hydrocephalus is understood as a deficit at cranial arachnoid villi and granulation absorption sites. However, there has been evidence that extracranial lymphatic vessels in the ethmoid bone region also play a role indicated by decreased lymphatic absorption in rat models of hydrocephalus. Treatment typically involves surgical shunt placement or endoscopic third ventriculostomy (ETV) technique with or without choroid plexus cauterization (CPC). These surgical interventions have high failure risks and complications that require re-intervention, further increasing morbidity and mortality risks. To date, there are few nonsurgical treatment strategies, but many have proved limited benefit, and many patients still require surgery. This analysis lays out the typical treatments and explores new, innovative interventions by highlighting the active role of brain parenchymal tissue in the pathogenesis of hydrocephalus.

Keywords: intracranial pressure, beta-integrins, choroid plexus, parenchymal pressure, ventricular pressure

1. Introduction

Hydrocephalus refers to cerebrospinal fluid (CSF) accumulation within cerebral ventricles [1]. The condition is most frequently seen in infants, secondary to congenital malformations and intraventricular hemorrhage observed in premature babies [1]. Studies have estimated that around 40% of primary hydrocephalus has a genetic basis [2, 3]. Additionally, pediatric hydrocephalus has a high incidence rate of approximately 0.1–0.6% of live births, likely due to intraventricular hemorrhage in premature infants [3, 4]. Nonetheless, posthemorrhagic hydrocephalus is not just in premature infants; it can also be seen in older populations due to the increased risk of stroke and other intensive brain injuries.

IntechOpen

However, the incidence rate of pediatric hydrocephalus is significantly higher in low-income countries because of an increased occurrence of neural tube defects and postinfectious hydrocephalus [5, 6]. Hydrocephalus incidence is 123 per 100,000 births in low-income countries versus 79 per 100,000 births in high-income countries, making it a common congenital defect globally [6]. The mortality rate of untreated hydrocephalus is high at around 20–87%, and treated hydrocephalus has a high cost of care due to work-up, treatment, equipment, follow-ups, and complication management [6]. With this high incidence rate, the largest disease burden in low-income countries, and the high cost of management compounded by death if left untreated, it is critical to continue understanding the pathophysiology and etiology behind hydrocephalus and use the knowledge to inform treatment. This paper discusses the traditional clinical treatment options for hydrocephalus and explores promising interventions informed by etiology. There are many complications associated with traditional treatment strategies; consequently, this review aims to understand the pathophysiology of hydrocephalus and draw connections between brain parenchymal tissue and hydrocephalus pathogenesis to explore future non-invasive interventions.

2. Methods

Articles were gathered using PubMed and Google Scholar. PubMed and Google Scholar search terms included: hydrocephalus clinical treatment, non-surgical hydrocephalus treatment, memantine hydrocephalus, acetazolamide hydrocephalus, prevalence of pediatric hydrocephalus, TRPV4 antagonist hydrocephalus, SPAK inhibitor hydrocephalus. There were no exclusion criteria regarding the type of article, as reviews, books, meta-analyses, clinical trials, and original studies were reviewed from any publication year. The pieces were reviewed for relevance to hydrocephalus and therapeutic approaches. This review will highlight etiology followed by pathophysiology, including the role of aquaporins, and the connection to clinical treatments. We will address problems with traditional surgical interventions. Lastly, we will highlight the non-surgical interventions used for hydrocephalus treatment, including acetazolamide, memantine, TRPV4 antagonist, NKCC1/SPAK inhibitors.

3. Etiology

Hydrocephalus is widely classified as communicating and non-communicating. Communicating hydrocephalus has no defect in CSF flow but rather is due to compromised CSF absorption with either over- or under-production of CSF. Communicating type hydrocephalus is classically caused by post-hemorrhagic or post-inflammatory changes, commonly subarachnoid hemorrhage or bacterial meningitis complications [1]. Communicating hydrocephalus has been mainly understood as a deficit at the cranial arachnoid villi and granulation absorption site. However, the literature has provided evidence for the role of extracranial lymphatic vessels located in the ethmoid bone region. It has been shown that lymphatic absorption is decreased in a rat animal model of hydrocephalus. On the other hand, non-communicating hydrocephalus arises due to intraventricular CSF obstruction. The obstruction is commonly at the foramen of Monro, to the aqueduct of Sylvius, the fourth ventricle, or the foramen magnum [1]. Non-communicating types can arise from hemorrhage, traumatic brain injury, brain tumor, cyst, or infection [7].

The CSF nourishes, protects, and removes toxic waste metabolites from the brain [1]. The leading production site of the CSF is the choroid plexus, with the cells connected via tight junctions. The blood-CSF barrier that forms protects the brain and serves as a shock absorber between the skull and the brain. Furthermore, CSF establishes homeostasis and composition consistency, facilitating proper neuronal functioning. This is an immune-privileged site and thus lacks substantial immunoglobulins. The central nervous system (CNS) immune cells, the microglial cells, are metabolically active and function to remove damaged or unused neuronal boutons [7].

4. Pathophysiology

As noted before, hydrocephalus is defined as excessive CSF in the brain. The choroid plexus produces CSF within the lateral, third, and fourth ventricles. The fluid travels from the choroid plexus in the lateral ventricle, through the ventricular system, through the foramen of Monro to the third ventricle, and into the fourth ventricle via cerebral aqueduct or aqueduct of Sylvius. The CSF leaves the fourth ventricle laterally through the foramen of Luschka or medially through the foramen of Magendie into the subarachnoid space. CSF that travels through the foramen of Luschka will go to the cisternal or cerebral cortex subarachnoid space. Disruption in the flow of CSF, either by a mass or via absorption defect, plays a key role in the pathogenesis of hydrocephalus.

4.1 Role of extracranial lymphatic vessels

CSF absorption primarily occurs at arachnoid granulations that protrude into dural venous sinuses, largely the superior sagittal sinus [1]. However, Nagra et al. [8] a previous study has provided evidence that extracranial lymphatic vessel plays a significant role in CSF absorption. Furthermore, impairment of CSF absorption at the level of extracranial lymphatic vessels results in hydrocephalus [7, 9].

Absorption pathways of CSF play a critical role in maintaining normal intracranial pressure. The primary pathway for CSF absorption is through arachnoid villi and then is directed into the superior sagittal sinus. These arachnoid villi can be thought of as finger-like projections extending into the venous sinus, allowing for CSF reabsorption into the bloodstream [10].

Emerging evidence through animal studies suggests that extracranial lymphatic vessels at ethmoid turbinates play a role in CSF absorption. Qualitatively, the use of India Ink in rat models demonstrates structural channels connecting the cribriform plate to the nasal submucosa [11]. Similarly, studies utilizing the murine model injected Evan's blue high-contrast tracers into the CSF fluid and demonstrated CSFs ability to permeate the nasal lymphatic system [12]. Sheep and rabbit studies using mathematical modeling and various tracers injected into the CSF, such as 131I Human Serum Albumin (HSA), India Ink, and Indigo Carmine, suggest that extracranial lymphatic vessels play a significant role in CSF drainage [11, 13, 14].

Through the use of yellow MicroFil injections, researchers demonstrated the connection between the subarachnoid space and nasal mucosa and turbinates in rat, pig, monkey, mice, and human cadaver studies [15]. Mathematical modeling has shown that 40–50% and greater than 50% of CSF drainage occurs through the olfactory pathway in rats, rabbits, and sheep, respectively [13, 14, 16]. While animal studies have shown extracranial lymphatic vessels at the ethmoid turbinates play a significant role in CSF absorption, further *in-vivo* studies in living humans are necessary. Human cadaver studies cannot accurately model the CSF fluid mechanics that occur in living beings.

With respect to this concept, there has been evidence that the outflow resistance of CSF is impaired globally in Kaolin rat models of communicating hydrocephalus. The decline in outflow resistance had a significant positive correlation to the severity of hydrocephalus, measured by an increased ventricular volume [10].

4.2 Role of aquaporins

Various studies have pointed toward aquaporin channels playing a role in hydrocephalus. Aquaporins (AQPs) are water channels that facilitate water movement across membranes. AQP1 and AQP4 play a role in CSF production and water removal from the brain and, thus, have been implicated in the development of hydrocephalus [17].

Mice experiments have shown that AQP1 is associated with CSF production and management of intracranial pressure [7]. Measurements done evaluating water permeability of the choroid plexus between wild-type and AQP1 null mice showed that AQP1 deletion leads to a five-fold decrease in the osmotic gradient of the ventricular membrane [18]. AQP1, which is located on the choroid plexus epithelium and plays a role in CSF production, has been implicated in the development of hydrocephalus using the kaolin-induced hydrocephalus model in mice [19]. Mice with kaolin-induced hydrocephalus demonstrated a 50% reduction of AQP1 by endocytic retrieval and reduced ventricular size of the AQP-1 null mice [19].

Furthermore, AQP4 is located at the astrocyte foot processes of the blood-brain barrier and glial cells of the brain parenchyma [20]. A rat study involving Sprague-Dawley rats demonstrated increased AQP4 expression after mild hydrocephalus induction with kaolin injection [21]. There was also increased AQP4 expression in congenital hydrocephalus Texas rats [21]. However, Wistar-Hannover rats demonstrated no change in AQP4 expression [22]. In humans, cortical brain biopsies in patients with chronic hydrocephalus showed increased AQP4 immunoreactivity compared to controls [7, 23]. The increase in AQP1 and AQP4 expression during hydrocephalus can be a compensatory mechanism to increase fluid clearance in the brain [20].

5. Surgical interventions

This section will discuss current surgical interventions, of which ventricular shunt placement is the gold-standard therapy.

5.1 Ventricular shunting

Traditionally, the gold standard treatment option for hydrocephalus involves the placement of a ventricular shunt that will redirect CSF flow to another part of the body for absorption [7]. The shunt is a ventricular catheter attached to a valve attached to a distal catheter [24]. The three most common shunts are ventriculoperitoneal, ventriculopleural, and ventriculoatrial, with the ventriculoperitoneal shunt most frequently used [25]. The ventriculoperitoneal shunt usually guides CSF from the lateral ventricle into the peritoneum. This shunt is advantageous in children as the distal peritoneal end can be left long and does not require adjustment as the child grows [1]. The ventriculoatrial shunt pushes CSF through the jugular vein and is then directed into the superior vena cava followed by the right atrium [1]. It is preferred for patients with peritonitis, extensive abdominal surgery, morbid obesity, or a history of ventriculoperitoneal shunt infection [1, 7]. Due to anatomical challenges requiring specialized surgical expertise, a ventriculopleural shunt is typically only used if the other shunt types fail [1].

5.2 Endoscopic third ventriculostomy (ETV)

However, shunting is not the only intervention in this class for hydrocephalus. An alternative to shunting is endoscopic third ventriculostomy (ETV). ETV involves opening the floor of the third ventricle to allow the accumulated CSF to enter the prepontine basal cistern [1, 7]. This is typically the procedure of choice for patients with aqueductal stenosis to avoid permanent shunt [1]. Certain risk factors have been identified that predispose to ETV failure, including young age, non-obstructive etiology, or shunt presence [4]. However, Zaben et al. [26] illuminates that even though there is a lower ETV success rate in lower age groups (44.4 vs. 66.7%), there is a comparable safety profile independent of age, thus indicating that ETV remains a viable option for infants 1 year or younger with obstructive hydrocephalus.

Additional research has been conducted exploring the viability of ETV with choroid plexus cauterization (CPC). CPC is an innovative approach introduced in 1910 and reinstated as a viable technique by Dr. Benjamin Warf [27]. In infants under one-year-old, Warf [27] demonstrated the utility of ETV with CPC to treat hydrocephalus. He illuminated that EVT/CPC was more successful than solely ETV in this age population and is a top choice for infants with non-post-infectious hydrocephalus or myelomeningocele. However, a meta-analysis [28] found no overall benefit to ETV/CPC versus ETV alone, but they did indicate that subgroup analysis demonstrated benefit in sub-Saharan African populations [28].

Furthermore, in 2020, the Hydrocephalus Clinical Research Network expanded on the research, revealing higher success rates for CSF shunt insertion (72% at 6 months and 65% at 12 months) than ETV/CPC (52% at 6 and 12 months) for infants in first-round hydrocephalus treatment [29]. About 3 to 5 years after the initial treatment, the ETV group showed fewer surgical revisions than those with CSF shunt insertion, but this was a non-statistically significant finding. Patients with ETV/CPC for the first treatment had higher mean hydrocephalus-related revision surgeries than those with ETV alone or CSF shunt insertion over the first year post-surgery. This group suggested a time-dependent benefit of ETV over CSF shunting [29].

Generally, these studies illuminate the need for further trials and studies to investigate the efficacy of CPC and ETV therapy in various patient populations and medically underserved areas and weigh the advantages and disadvantages.

5.3 Problems with traditional surgical interventions

It is important to note that permanent CSF interventions are often associated with a high failure risk and can involve re-intervention [4]. The risk of surgical infection is approximately 10%, and shunt failure rates are around 21–42% in the first year post-placement [30]. In the first 2 years, shunt failure in children can be at a frequency of up to 50% [4]. Furthermore, each shunt failure necessitates at least one additional operation, increasing morbidity and mortality risks [4]. Additionally, there is risk of shunt obstruction via flow blockage or infection due to biofilm formation, commonly seen with *Staphylococcus epidermidis* and *Staphylococcus aureus* [25, 31].

A recent case report [30] shared a successful first-in-human treatment with a miniature biomimetic transdural shunt. This novel minimally invasive endovascular shunt mimics the function of arachnoid granulation to filter CSF from the CNS into the intracranial venous sinus network. This valved shunt has transdural deployment at the inferior petrosal sinus. The typical reabsorption of CSF flow was restored through the cerebellopontine angle cistern to the inferior petrosal sinus. The team utilized this novel approach on one octogenarian (age range 80–89) patient with subarachnoid hemorrhage from a ruptured middle cerebral aneurysm. An external ventricular drain (EVD) was placed and showed decreased frontal and lateral horns and third ventricle size, as demonstrated through a post-procedure MRI. The imaging also showed normal venous blood flow through the inferior petrosal sinus and internal jugular vein around the implant. This successful catheter-based treatment is a major development in establishing a more simplistic, non-invasive surgical intervention for patients requiring shunting treatment. However, this was a first-in-human study, and thus, further testing is necessary to establish long-term efficacy, safety, and applicable patient population.

6. Non-surgical treatment

The following will talk about non-surgical interventions, most of which are still at the research level.

6.1 Acetazolamide

One frequently discussed treatment option for hydrocephalus is the carbonic anhydrase inhibitor, Acetazolamide [32]. The choroid plexus has high levels of carbonic anhydrase, so acetazolamide will directly inhibit CSF production [32]. However, studies have shown that the benefit of acetazolamide in hydrocephalic children is negligible [32].

Furthermore, there is high clinical certainty that the combination of acetazolamide and furosemide is not seen as a viable treatment option for posthemorrhagic hydrocephalus in infants [32, 33]. Two studies reported that preterm infants with posthemorrhagic hydrocephalus treated with dual therapy had a higher risk of neurological complications, morbidity, and mortality [33]. Additionally, the International Posthemorrhagic Ventricular Dilatation (PHVD) Drug Trial Group established increased rates of shunt placement in those treated with acetazolamide and furosemide and increased morbidity (84 vs. 60%) compared to the standard approach [33, 34].

However, in adults, acetazolamide was used instead of shunting, and it decreased intracranial pressure in cases of Normal Pressure Hydrocephalus (NPH), a type of communicating hydrocephalus [7]. Moreover, it has been established as a good predictor of shunting response in NPH patients [35].

6.2 Memantine

More recently, memantine has become a drug of discussion surrounding hydrocephalus treatment. Memantine is a selective, non-competitive antagonist of the N-methyl-D-aspartate (NMDA) receptor, which has a neuroprotective contribution in neurological disease [36, 37]. A previous study [36] explored the role of memantine therapy on neurologic and behavioral outcomes in kaolin-induced hydrocephalus rats. Memantine therapy stabilized ventricular enlargement with some behavioral improvement but did not reduce brain tissue changes.

Another team [37] explored the neuroprotective effect of memantine in hydrocephalus-induced Wistar rats treated with or without a ventricular-subcutaneous shunt. Memantine treatment had significant improvement in sensorimotor development, spatial memory preservation, and astrocytic reaction reduction in corpus callosum, cortex and germinal matrix. When memantine was treated with shunt placement, there was a reduction in the cell death cascade. There is a promising response with memantine treatment that has the potential to assist in hydrocephalus treatment with or without other procedures, but more research must be completed.

6.3 TRPV4 antagonist

Transient receptor potential vanilloid 4 (TRPV4) is a nonselective, Ca^{2+}-permeable channel expressed in the choroid plexus and facilitates ion flow across the epithelial membrane, influencing water movement and CSF production. It is known as a hub protein as it is activated by and integrates many stimuli. TRPV4 can be activated chemically via inflammatory mediators (arachidonic acid metabolites or cytokines) or physically via mechanical (pressure) and osmotic changes–mechanisms also known to cause hydrocephalus.

A study utilizing a genetic rat model of communicating hydrocephalus showed that two different TRPV4 antagonists inhibited ventriculomegaly development [38]. Their data supported the relationship between TRPV4 and hydrocephalus development from cell surface expression or activation changes. Furthermore, the TRPV4 antagonists did not change ventricular volumes in normal animals and thus were mainly applicable in the hydrocephalic rats. Through the role of TRPV4 in regulating transepithelial ion flux and cell permeability in the choroid plexus, there is the possible utility of TRPV4 antagonists for most forms of hydrocephalus. Still, the idea of TRPV4 antagonist as a treatment measure is a new idea that requires much further examination due to multiple compounding factors, including electrolyte balance and fluid flux complexities.

Furthermore, Toft-Bertelsen et al. [39] demonstrated lysophosphatidic acid (LPA) elevation in patients with subarachnoid hemorrhage and intraventricular hemorrhage-induced rat models. Elevated LPA directly impacted TRPV4, which activates the WNK/SPAK signaling path that promotes NKCC1-mediated CSF hypersecretion and ventricular enlargement. SPAK is a highly expressed kinase in the choroid plexus and a vital regulator of NKCC1. It was concluded that LPA is a lipid agonist of TRPV4 that facilitates the SPAK and NKCC1 pathway leading to increased CSF secretion. This fundamental knowledge suggests the need for additional studies on potential therapies targeting LPA, TRPV4, SPAK, or NKCC1 to reduce hydrocephalus.

6.4 NKCC1 and SPAK inhibitors

The above discussion of TRPV4 and NKCC1 indicates their roles in maintaining CSF volume homeostasis and composition during disease states. While TRPV4 is activated due to osmotic changes, pressure, or inflammatory mediators, NKCC1 is activated by changes in electrolyte concentration. Furthermore, while different kinases activate TRPV4, NKCC1 is triggered primarily by WNK-SPAK and maintains cell volume levels and CSF composition [3].

One study [40] showed that NKCC1 phosphorylation in choroid plexus epithelium facilitates CSF hypersecretion by the NLRP3 inflammasome process. As part of the innate immune system, the NLRP3 inflammasome has been connected to neuroinflammation, and this study illuminated its function in hydrocephalus pathogenesis.

Furthermore, Zhang et al. [41] designed and synthesized a non-ATP-competitive SPAK inhibitor called ZT-1a. This drug is unique in its development as the team used a "scaffold-hybrid" strategy, combining the pharmacophores from previously developed SPAK inhibitors (Closantel, Rafoxanide, and STOCK1S-14,279). ZT-1a disrupted SPAK interaction with WNK, inhibited NKCC1 activity, and decreased CSF hypersecretion in post-hemorrhagic hydrocephalus models. With further study, this exciting innovation has strong therapeutic potential for hydrocephalus.

6.5 Potential for extracranial lymphatic vessels

As noted, extracranial lymphatics play a crucial role in absorbing CSF. In the rat model of hydrocephalus, extracranial lymphatic vessel absorption was decreased. With respect to this, a study that used a sheep hindlimb model observed the emergence of lymphedema following the removal of popliteal lymph nodes [42]. Similarly, Baker et al. induced lymphedema by excising a single popliteal lymph node along with its associated vessels [43]. About this, after inducing the lymph edema, this Johnston's group showed that an autologous lymph node transplantation lowered the lymph edema significantly. This is indirect evidence that enhancing lymphatic absorption can be used as a therapeutic strategy to deal with different pathologies.

Studies by Brunner et al. [44] demonstrate the importance of signaling molecules in lymphangiogenesis [45]. Specifically, their studies showed that VEGF-C to VEGFR3 modulates lymphatic vessel growth, particularly in the restructuring of the diabetic wound matrix. Interestingly, the use of viral vectors to increase VEGF-C expression can improve both lymphatic and blood vessel growth.

Furthermore, Choi et al. [46] showed that 9-cis Retinoic Acid can be applied therapeutically to facilitate lymphangiogenesis and lymphatic restoration.

Applying this concept to the brain, substances such as VEGF-C/VEGFR3 and 9-cis Retinoic Acid can enhance the lymphatic uptake of the fluid and if used locally can induce lymphangiogenesis at the ethmoid bone level to help alleviate hydrocephalus.

7. Discussion

Hydrocephalus, marked by ventricular expansion due to CSF accumulation, has a high burden of disease and cost of treatment that further accumulates with the high complication risks associated with the current standard of treatment. Management of this condition involves deviation of CSF with lumboperitoneal or ventriculoperitoneal shunts or the ETV technique. Placing a shunt in the brain through mini-laparotomy surgery can result in neurological complications, incisional abdominal herniation, and CSF pseudocyst formation [9]. Shunts provide symptomatic improvement, but one must consider the significant number of debilitating neurological deficits, high revision rates, mechanical failures, and infections, making this a poor treatment standard [9].

Nagra G's thesis challenges the traditional view of hydrocephalus as a plumbing issue by drawing critical conclusions concerning the etiology of hydrocephalus which can revolutionize hydrocephalus treatment [10]. With respect to this, the very conflict of accepting the textbook definition of CSF absorption via arachnoid villi and granulation was challenged. This was done by providing quantitative experimental data supporting extracranial lymphatic vessels' role at discrete anatomical locations. The CSF absorption impairment of these vessels contributes to hydrocephalus. Specifically, using the kaolin rat model of hydrocephalus, CSF outflow resistance was increased, and absorption was shown to be significantly decreased. Furthermore, to understand the molecular mechanical property of ventricular brain expansion, the Nagra et al. [47] study illustrated that β1-integrin and extracellular matrix interactions actively regulate interstitial fluid pressure. Any disruption to those interactions decreases brain parenchymal fluid pressure with respect to ventricles, creating a pressure gradient that leads to ventricular expansion.

Nagra et al. [47] employed a micropipette servo-null pressure measuring system to investigate the active role of brain parenchyma in inducing ventriculomegaly. Two sets of experiments were conducted: one focused on measuring pressure in the lateral ventricle and adjacent parenchymal tissue before and after continuous injection of beta-integrin blocking antibodies using a servo-nulling pressure measuring system. The second set involved injecting beta-integrin blocking antibodies into the brain and assessing ventriculomegaly by brain sectioning after 2 weeks. The results showed a decline in periventricular pressures relative to pre-injection values when antibodies to beta-1 integrins were injected, whereas ventricular pressures were elevated and significantly higher than periventricular interstitial pressures. The estimated ventricular to periventricular pressure gradients reached up to 4.3 cm H_2O. In chronic preparations, enlarged ventricles were observed in 72% of animals receiving anti-integrin antibodies but not in those receiving isotype control antibodies. This led to the conclusion that disrupting beta-1 integrin-matrix interactions generates pressure gradients favoring ventricular expansion, providing a plausible mechanism for hydrocephalus development [47].

This concept was formulated after considering that injecting anti-beta-1 integrin antibodies into the skin simulates inflammatory effects, leading to a significant drop in interstitial fluid pressure [48]. Although various causes and inflammatory mediators consistently induce this effect, what was particularly relevant to the Nagra et al. [47] study is that the injection of antibodies targeting alpha-2-beta-1 or beta-1 integrins can lower interstitial fluid pressure, indicating their key role in regulating this phenomenon [49]. This suggests that the interstitial matrix is dynamic and disrupting its integrity can modify tissue pressure. Applying this concept to the brain, my group proposed that disturbances in beta-1 integrin function could be one of the defining factors leading to ventriculomegaly and offered a new perspective on hydrocephalus development.

Articulating the former, Nagra G proposed the hypothesis that the extracellular matrix actively regulates interstitial fluid pressure rather than merely participating passively. Their data suggests that matrix components within the brain parenchyma exhibit similar dynamics to those observed in peripheral tissue function. Beta-1 integrins are believed to play crucial roles in central nervous system function and are expressed in choroidal and ependymal cells, glial cells, and vascular structures throughout the neuropil [50–52]. Astrocyte fibers, which surround particular microvessels in the adult primate, also express beta-1 integrins, as do the endothelial cells themselves [52]. Reduction of beta-1 integrin expression, specifically in neuronal and glial precursors, has been associated with convoluted cortex and reduced brain size [53]. Additionally, humans and mice with mutations in the laminin alpha-2 chain, an essential ligand for beta-1 integrins, exhibit disorganized cerebral cortices and ventricular dilation [54–56]. These findings suggest that disruption of beta-1 integrin-laminin interactions may contribute to pressure patterns and the development of hydrocephalus.

It is worth noting that dystroglycan, another receptor sharing laminin as a primary matrix ligand with several beta-1 integrin receptors, has been associated with ventriculomegaly in dystroglycan-null mice [57]. The authors speculated that this might result from dysfunction of arachnoid granulations or stenosis of the cerebral aqueduct. However, it is plausible that the loss of dystroglycan specifically in epiblasts could affect cell-matrix interactions similarly to the injection of beta-1 integrin antibodies.

Understanding this etiology is useful when considering therapeutics useful for hydrocephalus treatment that can improve outcomes and limit side effects. It has been shown experimentally that decreased tissue pressure in the skin can be reversed with the anti-inflammatory agent α-trinositol [58, 59]. Platelet-derived growth factor (PDGF-BB) isoform also can play a role by counteracting edema development through stimulation of αVβ3-integrins activity and adjusting extracellular matrix tension [60, 61]. If these themes prove relevant to brain physiology, these could be valuable avenues of pharmacological treatment for hydrocephalus.

Studies using magnetic resonance elastography (MRE) and diffusion tensor imaging (DTI) have provided quantitative data on brain tissue mechanics and support a decrease in compliance forces in a hydrocephalic brain and is proportional to the hydrocephalus severity [62, 63]. Nagra et al. [47] demonstrated the role of integrin-matrix interactions in the development of hydrocephalus. Further, the data from human MRE and DTI studies hold up the experimental matrix integrity disruption concept [62]. Going forward, there is utility in exploring the role of anti-inflammatory agents, such as a-trinositol, or PDGF-BB, in individuals with hydrocephalus or post-shunt placement showing symptom improvement improving the extracellular matrix damage. Building upon MRE and DTI data and experimental support for matrix disorganization, Nagra proposed investigating whether administering these therapeutic agents to children with hydrocephalus or following shunt insertion could alleviate symptoms and reverse matrix damage. This hypothesis could be tested using imaging modalities, and it is anticipated that MRE and DTI data would show improvement in children receiving these agents. If successful, this approach could lead to the development of pharmacological treatments for hydrocephalus, reducing dependence on shunts.

8. Conclusion

This paper shares the currently accepted and utilized techniques for hydrocephalus. Also, it discusses a shift in the understanding of hydrocephalus from a purely plumbing problem to an active involvement of the brain matrix in creating pressure gradients. The disruption of beta-1 integrin-matrix interactions and the resulting pressure gradients are proposed as key factors contributing to ventriculomegaly. These findings can help reduce the need for expensive, invasive, and, in some instances, hard-to-access therapies. By opening up new avenues for potential therapeutic interventions and raising the possibility of treating hydrocephalus with pharmacological agents, there is a potential for the reduced need for shunts. With high incidence rates, with most significant numbers in low-income countries, and elevated mortality rate if left untreated, there is an increased need for more accessible, lower-cost treatment plans based on mechanisms of hydrocephalus. There is still much to be explored regarding hydrocephalus's risk factors, etiology, and pathophysiology. Further research and clinical trials are required to validate these hypotheses and determine their clinical applicability. As studies expand, the gained knowledge must be considered and inform future treatment with a goal of decreased invasiveness, complications, and cost. We aspire to leverage the synergistic potential of lymphatic vessels combined with shunt therapy to alleviate the pathology of hydrocephalus.

Acknowledgements

We would like to acknowledge Dr. Miles Johnston of University of Toronto, Canada for his knowledge and work at Sunnybrook Health Centre.

Conflict of interest

The authors declare no conflict of interest.

Author details

Sarah Arianna Mirkhaef, Lauren Harbaugh and Gurjit Nagra*
Arkansas College of Osteopathic Medicine, Fort Smith, Arkansas, United States

*Address all correspondence to: gurjit.nagra09@gmail.com

References

[1] Koleva M, De Jesus O. Hydrocephalus. Treasure Island (FL): StatPearls Publishing; 2023. Available from: http://www.ncbi.nlm.nih.gov/books/NBK560875/ [Accessed: May 19, 2023]

[2] Zhang J, Williams MA, Rigamonti D. Genetics of human hydrocephalus. Journal of Neurology. 2006;**253**(10):1255-1266

[3] Blazer-Yost BL. Consideration of kinase inhibitors for the treatment of hydrocephalus. International Journal of Molecular Sciences. 2023;**24**(7):6673

[4] Hochstetler A, Raskin J, Blazer-Yost BL. Hydrocephalus: Historical analysis and considerations for treatment. European Journal of Medical Research. 2022;**27**(1):168

[5] Dewan MC, Rattani A, Mekary R, Glancz LJ, Yunusa I, Baticulon RE, et al. Global hydrocephalus epidemiology and incidence: Systematic review and meta-analysis. Journal of Neurosurgery. 2018;**130**:1065-1079

[6] Enslin JMN, Thango NS, Figaji A, Fieggen GA. Hydrocephalus in low and middle-income countries-progress and challenges. Neurology India. 2021;**69**(8):292

[7] Agyei AA, Miles JD, Nagra G. Rethinking hydrocephalus via interventional pathophysiology. In: Campbell RD, editor. Hydrocephalus: From Diagnosis to Treatment. New York: Nova Science Publishers; 2021. (Neurology–Laboratory and Clinical Research Developments)

[8] Nagra G, Koh L, Zakharov A, Armstrong D, Johnston M. Quantification of cerebrospinal fluid transport across the cribriform plate into lymphatics in rats. American Journal of Physiology-Regulatory, Integrative and Comparative Physiology. 2006;**291**(5):R1383-R1389

[9] Nagra G, Wagshul ME, Rashid S, Li J, McAllister JP, Johnston M. Elevated CSF outflow resistance associated with impaired lymphatic CSF absorption in a rat model of kaolin-induced communicating hydrocephalus. Fluids and Barriers of the CNS. 2010;**7**(1):4

[10] Nagra G. Extracellular Fluid Systems in the Brain and the Pathogenesis of Hydrocephalus. University of Toronto [Internet]; 2010; Available from: https://tspace.library.utoronto.ca/bitstream/1807/26309/5/Nagra_Gurjit_201011_PhD_thesis.pdf

[11] Kida S, Pantazis A, Weller RO. CSF drains directly from the subarachnoid space into nasal lymphatics in the rat. Anatomy, histology and immunological significance. Neuropathology and Applied Neurobiology. 1993;**19**(6):480-488

[12] Norwood JN, Zhang Q, Card D, Craine A, Ryan TM, Drew PJ. Anatomical basis and physiological role of cerebrospinal fluid transport through the murine cribriform plate. eLife. 2019;**8**:e44278

[13] Boulton M, Flessner M, Armstrong D, Hay J, Johnston M. Lymphatic drainage of the CNS: Effects of lymphatic diversion/ligation on CSF protein transport to plasma. The American Journal of Physiology. 1997;**272**(5 Pt 2):R1613-R1619

[14] Boulton M, Flessner M, Armstrong D, Mohamed R, Hay J, Johnston M. Contribution of extracranial

lymphatics and arachnoid villi to the clearance of a CSF tracer in the rat. The American Journal of Physiology. 1999;**276**(3):R818-R823

[15] Johnston M, Zakharov A, Papaiconomou C, Salmasi G, Armstrong D. Evidence of connections between cerebrospinal fluid and nasal lymphatic vessels in humans, non-human primates and other mammalian species. Cerebrospinal Fluid Research. 2004;**1**(1):2

[16] Silver I, Kim C, Mollanji R, Johnston M. Cerebrospinal fluid outflow resistance in sheep: Impact of blocking cerebrospinal fluid transport through the cribriform plate. Neuropathology and Applied Neurobiology. 2002;**28**(1):67-74

[17] Carbrey JM, Agre P. Discovery of the Aquaporins and development of the field. In: Beitz E, editor. Aquaporins [Internet]. Berlin, Heidelberg: Springer Berlin Heidelberg; 2009. pp. 3-28. (Hofmann F, editor. Handbook of Experimental Pharmacology; vol. 190). Available from: http://link.springer.com/10.1007/978-3-540-79885-9_1 [Accessed: June 3, 2023]

[18] Oshio K, Watanabe H, Song Y, Verkman AS, Manley GT. Reduced cerebrospinal fluid production and intracranial pressure in mice lacking choroid plexus water channel Aquaporin-1. The FASEB Journal. 2005;**19**(1):76-78

[19] Wang D, Nykanen M, Yang N, Winlaw D, North K, Verkman AS, et al. Altered cellular localization of aquaporin-1 in experimental hydrocephalus in mice and reduced ventriculomegaly in aquaporin-1 deficiency. Molecular and Cellular Neuroscience. 2011;**46**(1):318-324

[20] Verkman AS, Tradtrantip L, Smith AJ, Yao X. Aquaporin water channels and hydrocephalus. Pediatric Neurosurgery. 2017;**52**(6):409-416

[21] Paul L, Madan M, Rammling M, Chigurupati S, Chan SL, Pattisapu JV. Expression of aquaporin 1 and 4 in a congenital hydrocephalus rat model. Neurosurgery. 2011;**68**(2):462-473

[22] Aghayev K, Bal E, Rahimli T, Mut M, Balcı S, Vrionis F, et al. Aquaporin-4 expression is not elevated in mild hydrocephalus. Acta Neurochirurgica. 2012;**154**(4):753-759

[23] Skjolding AD, Rowland IJ, Søgaard LV, Praetorius J, Penkowa M, Juhler M. Hydrocephalus induces dynamic spatiotemporal regulation of aquaporin-4 expression in the rat brain. Fluids and Barriers of the CNS. 2010;**7**(1):20

[24] Fowler JB, De Jesus O, Mesfin FB. Ventriculoperitoneal Shunt [Internet]. Treasure Island (FL): StatPearls Publishing; 2023 Available from: https://www.ncbi.nlm.nih.gov/books/NBK459351/

[25] Hanak BW, Bonow RH, Harris CA, Browd SR. Cerebrospinal fluid shunting complications in children. Pediatric Neurosurgery. 2017;**52**(6):381-400

[26] Zaben M, Manivannan S, Sharouf F, Hammad A, Patel C, Bhatti I, et al. The efficacy of endoscopic third ventriculostomy in children 1 year of age or younger: A systematic review and meta-analysis. European Journal of Paediatric Neurology. 2020;**26**:7-14

[27] Warf BC. Comparison of endoscopic third ventriculostomy alone and combined with choroid plexus cauterization in infants younger than 1 year of age: A prospective study in 550 African children. Journal of Neurosurgery: Pediatrics. 2005;**103**(6):475-481

[28] Ellenbogen Y, Brar K, Yang K, Lee Y, Ajani O. Comparison of endoscopic third ventriculostomy with or without choroid plexus cauterization in pediatric hydrocephalus: A systematic review and meta-analysis. Journal of Neurosurgery: Pediatrics. 2020;**26**(4):371-378

[29] Pindrik J, Riva-Cambrin J, Kulkarni AV, Alvey JS, Reeder RW, Pollack IF, et al. Surgical resource utilization after initial treatment of infant hydrocephalus: Comparing ETV, early experience of ETV with choroid plexus cauterization, and shunt insertion in the hydrocephalus clinical research network. Journal of Neurosurgery: Pediatrics. 2020;**26**(4):337-345

[30] Lylyk P, Lylyk I, Bleise C, Scrivano E, Lylyk PN, Beneduce B, et al. First-in-human endovascular treatment of hydrocephalus with a miniature biomimetic transdural shunt. Journal of Neuro Interventional Surgery. 2022;**14**(5):495-499

[31] Gutierrez-Murgas Y, Snowden JN. Ventricular shunt infections: Immunopathogenesis and clinical management. Journal of Neuroimmunology. 2014;**276**(1-2):1-8

[32] Del Bigio MR, Di Curzio DL. Nonsurgical therapy for hydrocephalus: A comprehensive and critical review. Fluids and Barriers of the CNS. 2015;**13**(1):3

[33] Mazzola CA, Choudhri AF, Auguste KI, Limbrick DD, Rogido M, Mitchell L, et al. Pediatric hydrocephalus: Systematic literature review and evidence-based guidelines. Part 2: Management of posthemorrhagic hydrocephalus in premature infants. Journal of Neurosurgery Pediatrics. 2014;**14**(Supplement_1):8-23

[34] International PHVD Drug Trail Group. International randomised controlled trial of acetazolamide and furosemide in posthaemorrhagic ventricular dilatation in infancy. International PHVD drug trial group. Lancet. 1998;**352**(9126):433-440

[35] Miyake H, Ohta T, Kajimoto Y, Deguchi J. Diamox® challenge test to decide indications for cerebrospinal fluid shunting in normal pressure hydrocephalus. Acta Neurochirurgica. 1999;**141**(11):1187-1193

[36] Di Curzio DL, Nagra G, Mao X, Del Bigio MR. Memantine treatment of juvenile rats with kaolin-induced hydrocephalus. Brain Research. 2018;**1689**:54-62

[37] Beggiora PDS, Da Silva SC, Rodrigues KP, Almeida TADL, Sampaio GB, Silva GAPDM, et al. Memantine associated with ventricular-subcutaneous shunt promotes behavioral improvement, reduces reactive astrogliosis and cell death in juvenile hydrocephalic rats. Journal of Chemical Neuroanatomy. 2022;**125**:102165

[38] Hochstetler AE, Smith HM, Preston DC, Reed MM, Territo PR, Shim JW, et al. TRPV4 antagonists ameliorate ventriculomegaly in a rat model of hydrocephalus. JCI Insight. 2020;**5**(18):e137646

[39] Toft-Bertelsen TL, Barbuskaite D, Heerfordt EK, Lolansen SD, Andreassen SN, Rostgaard N, et al. Lysophosphatidic acid as a CSF lipid in posthemorrhagic hydrocephalus that drives CSF accumulation via TRPV4-induced hyperactivation of NKCC1. Fluids and Barriers of the CNS. 2022;**19**(1):69

[40] Zhang Z, Tan Q, Guo P, Huang S, Jia Z, Liu X, et al. NLRP3 inflammasome-mediated choroid plexus hypersecretion contributes to hydrocephalus after

intraventricular hemorrhage via phosphorylated NKCC1 channels. Journal of Neuroinflammation. 2022;**19**(1):163

[41] Zhang J, Bhuiyan MIH, Zhang T, Karimy JK, Wu Z, Fiesler VM, et al. Modulation of brain cation-Cl– cotransport via the SPAK kinase inhibitor ZT-1a. Nature Communications. 2020;**11**:78

[42] Tobbia D, Semple J, Baker A, Dumont D, Semple A, Johnston M. Lymphedema development and lymphatic function following lymph node excision in sheep. Journal of Vascular Research. 2009;**46**(5):426-434

[43] Baker A, Kim H, Semple JL, Dumont D, Shoichet M, Tobbia D, et al. Experimental assessment of pro-lymphangiogenic growth factors in the treatment of post-surgical lymphedema following lymphadenectomy. Breast Cancer Research. 2010;**12**(5):R70

[44] Brunner LM, He Y, Cousin N, Scholl J, Albin LK, Schmucki B, et al. Promotion of lymphangiogenesis by targeted delivery of VEGF-C improves diabetic wound healing. Cell. 2023;**12**(3):472

[45] Shimizu Y, Che Y, Murohara T. Therapeutic lymphangiogenesis is a promising strategy for secondary lymphedema. International Journal of Molecular Sciences. 2023;**24**(9):7774

[46] Choi I, Lee S, Kyoung Chung H, Suk Lee Y, Eui Kim K, Choi D, et al. 9-cis retinoic acid promotes lymphangiogenesis and enhances lymphatic vessel regeneration. Circulation. 2012;**125**(7):872-882

[47] Nagra G, Koh L, Aubert I, Kim M, Johnston M. Intraventricular injection of antibodies to β1-integrins generates pressure gradients in the brain favoring hydrocephalus development in rats. American Journal of Physiology-Regulatory, Integrative and Comparative Physiology. 2009;**297**(5):R1312-R1321

[48] Wiig H, Rubin K, Reed RK. New and active role of the interstitium in control of interstitial fluid pressure: Potential therapeutic consequences: Active control of interstitial fluid pressure. Acta Anaesthesiologica Scandinavica. 2003;**47**(2):111-121

[49] Reed RK, Rubin K, Wiig H, Rodt SA. Blockade of beta 1-integrins in skin causes edema through lowering of interstitial fluid pressure. Circulation Research. 1992;**71**(4):978-983

[50] Grooms SY, Terracio L, Jones LS. Anatomical localization of β1 integrin-like immunoreactivity in rat brain. Experimental Neurology. 1993;**122**(2):253-259

[51] Paulus W, Baur I, Schuppan D, Roggendorf W. Characterization of integrin receptors in normal and neoplastic human brain. The American Journal of Pathology. 1993;**143**(1):154-163

[52] Del Zoppo GJ, Milner R. Integrin–matrix interactions in the cerebral microvasculature. ATVB. 2006;**26**(9):1966-1975

[53] Graus-Porta D, Blaess S, Senften M, Littlewood-Evans A, Damsky C, Huang Z, et al. β1-class integrins regulate the development of laminae and folia in the cerebral and cerebellar cortex. Neuron. 2001;**31**(3):367-379

[54] Sunada Y, Edgar TS, Lotz BP, Rust RS, Campbell KP. Merosin-negative congenital muscular dystrophy associated with extensive brain abnormalities. Neurology. 1995;**45**(11):2084-2089

[55] Philpot J, Cowan F, Pennock J, Sewry C, Dubowitz V, Bydder G, et al. Merosin-deficient congenital muscular dystrophy: The spectrum of brain involvement on magnetic resonance imaging. Neuromuscular Disorders. 1999;**9**(2):81-85

[56] Miyagoe-Suzuki Y, Nakagawa M, Takeda S. Merosin and congenital muscular dystrophy. Microscopy Research and Technique. 2000;**48**(3-4):181-191

[57] Satz JS, Barresi R, Durbeej M, Willer T, Turner A, Moore SA, et al. Brain and eye malformations resembling Walker-Warburg syndrome are recapitulated in mice by dystroglycan deletion in the epiblast. The Journal of Neuroscience. 2008;**28**(42):10567-10575

[58] Lund T, Reed RK. Alpha-trinositol inhibits edema generation and albumin extravasation in thermally injured skin. Journal of Trauma and Acute Care Surgery. 1994;**36**(6):761

[59] Rodt SA, Reed RK, Ljungström M, Gustafsson TO, Rubin K. The anti-inflammatory agent alpha-trinositol exerts its edema-preventing effects through modulation of beta 1 integrin function. Circulation Research. 1994;**75**(5):942-948

[60] Rodt SA, Ahlén K, Berg A, Rubin K, Reed RK. A novel physiological function for platelet-derived growth factor-BB in rat dermis. The Journal of Physiology. 1996;**495**(Pt. 1):193-200

[61] Lidén Å, Berg A, Nedrebø T, Reed RK, Rubin K. Platelet-derived growth factor BB–mediated normalization of dermal interstitial fluid pressure after mast cell degranulation depends on β3 but not β1 integrins. Circulation Research. 2006;**98**(5):635-641

[62] Tan K, Meiri A, Mowrey WB, Abbott R, Goodrich JT, Sandler AL, et al. Diffusion tensor imaging and ventricle volume quantification in patients with chronic shunt-treated hydrocephalus: A matched case-control study. Journal of Neurosurgery. 2018;**129**(6):1611-1622

[63] Aunan-Diop JS, Pedersen CB, Halle B, Jensen U, Munthe S, Harbo F, et al. Magnetic resonance elastography in normal pressure hydrocephalus—A scoping review. Neurosurgical Review. 2022;**45**(2):1157-1169

Chapter 3

Clinical Aspects in Which Symptoms May Indicate Cerebrospinal Fluid (CSF) Analysis

Mariana-Alis Neagoe

Abstract

This chapter aims to describe clinical aspects in which examination of cerebrospinal fluid is essential for diagnosis. Clinical signs and symptoms that may indicate analysis of cerebrospinal fluid may include changes in mental status, severe headache, difficulty speaking, difficulty walking, dizziness, fever, muscle weakness, sensitivity to light, and seizures. Cerebrospinal fluid is frequently collected by lumbar puncture—a procedure of mainly diagnostic value. Examination of the cerebrospinal fluid determines the appearance, chemical and cytological composition, and pressure. In some conditions, analysis of cerebrospinal fluid is no longer necessary to establish the diagnosis, but the presence of changes in cerebrospinal fluid increases the level of "comfort" for diagnosis. Today, the lumbar puncture is no longer used to examine all types of central nervous system disorders. However, it is still used to diagnose central nervous system infections, neuroimmunological disorders, tumours, Guillain-Barré syndrome, and multiple sclerosis.

Keywords: cerebrospinal fluid, central nervous system infections, headache, multiple sclerosis, polyradiculoneuritis

1. Introduction

This chapter aims to describe clinical aspects in which examination of cerebrospinal fluid is essential for diagnosis.

Clinical signs and symptoms that may indicate analysis of cerebrospinal fluid may include changes in mental status, severe headache, difficulty speaking, difficulty walking, dizziness, fever, muscle weakness, sensitivity to light, and seizures.

Cerebrospinal fluid is frequently collected by a lumbar puncture—a procedure of mainly diagnostic value.

Examination of the cerebrospinal fluid determines the appearance, chemical and cytological composition, and pressure.

In some conditions, analysis of cerebrospinal fluid is no longer necessary to establish the diagnosis, but the presence of changes in cerebrospinal fluid increases the level of "comfort" for diagnosis.

CSF examination is important for the differential diagnosis of a range of central nervous system (CNS) infections, meningitis, encephalitis, as well as subarachnoid haemorrhage, confusional states, acute stroke, status epilepticus, meningeal neoplasms, demyelinating diseases and vasculitis [1].

CSF examination—LP should be preceded by imaging examination. Given the high cost of neuroimaging exploration, the American College of Emergency Physicians (ACEP), following a comprehensive review of the literature in 2002, makes the following recommendation (level C): 'Adult headache patients with signs of intracranial hypertension (ICH), papillary oedema, absence of venous pulsations on ophthalmoscopic examination, altered mental status or focal neurological signs should be investigated initially by computer tomography (CT)'. The absence of signs of ICH allows a puncture without CT [2].

LP is recommended when suspected:

- Meningitis/encephalitis, subarachnoid haemorrhage (SAH), lymphomatosis, meningeal carcinomatosis,
- CSF pressure abnormalities that may be responsible for headache:
  - Pressure drop, below 90 mm H2O, post-traumatic brain injury (TBI) or LP,
  - increased pressure, above 200-250 mm H2O in idiopathic ICH, intracranial expansive processes, infectious processes, or intracranial haemorrhage.
- Suspicion of SAH even with normal CT requires LP with CSF examination. Fluid obtained by LP certifies the diagnosis of SAH if, being haemorrhagic, it shows a xanthochromic supernatant.
- In blood dyscrasias, LP may be performed when the platelet count is above 50,000/mmc [2].

2. Contents

2.1 Clinical signs and symptoms suggestive of CSF analysis are

2.1.1 Headache

Headaches are among the most common complaints of patients presenting to primary care and neurology and account for approximately 2% of all emergency department visits [3].

Because of its myriad potential causes, from benign to catastrophic, headache presents the clinician with a number of diagnostic and therapeutic challenges [3].

The results of the history and physical examination dictate appropriate diagnostic evaluations [3].

Faced with a patient with headache, the major clinical responsibility is to rule out structural or dynamic causes. Any expansive brain lesion can cause headache [1].

Headache characteristics of ICH. The location of the pain is not specific, although when a progressive headache begins at the back of the neck, herniation of the cerebellar tonsils is imminent. Headache is:

a. more pronounced in the morning;

b. aggravated by sitting or standing and improved by clinostatism;

c. aggravated by coughing, sneezing and vomiting;

d. relieved by aspirin or paracetamol in the early stages (in contrast to psychogenic headache);

e. associated with vomiting and eventually with papillary oedema and progressive focal signs. In the stuporous stage with hemiplegia and a mydriatic pupil (Hutchinson's) the diagnosis is late [1].

Sudden-onset headache occurs in TBI, spontaneous intracranial haemorrhages, hydrocephalus or meningeal irritation at any age, the elderly not being immune. The most common cause is acute meningeal irritation due to SAH or bacterial or viral (rarely fungal or malignant) meningitis. An abrupt onset with fever, headache and Kernig's sign accompanies severe headache, vomiting and photophobia. CSF analysis is mandatory if an infection is considered but after ruling out a brain abscess, tumour or haematoma [1].

LP is mandatory in cases of possible SAH (when neuroimaging alone is 99% sensitive), infectious or eosinophilic meningoencephalitis or pseudotumor cerebri. CSF is analysed for cells, protein, glucose, culture, cytology or special tests when warranted. In cases of possible haemorrhage, CSF should be centrifuged to detect the presence of xanthochromia. Opening pressure is compensated for in any patient with headache which does LP [3].

2.1.2 Changes in mental state

CNS dysfunctions (either decreased functioning leading to obnubilation and eventually coma, or reverse—hyperactivity leading to delirium) may be due to a primary neurological condition or may be secondary to a medical condition. Determining the patient's initial (baseline) mental status is crucial for identifying mild mental status disorders. More severe disturbances have more obvious presentations, but in all cases, from mild to severe, the clinical history of onset, progression and coexisting features are essential to identify the underlying cause [3].

Consciousness is the ability of the individual in a vigilant state to realise his or her own existence and that of the environment and to have adequate perception and responsiveness. Consciousness is an active process with multiple components, including attention, memory, motivation, abstract thinking and the performance of actions with different purposes [4].

In the physiology of the nervous system, two important properties of consciousness are described: (1) the level of consciousness, which quantitatively estimates perception, reactivity and alertness status, and (2) the content of consciousness, which qualitatively estimates perception and reactivity [4].

Pathological alterations in consciousness may result from damage to the nervous system or metabolic disturbances caused by systemic diseases. Consciousness is clinically assessed by testing the patient's ability to respond to sensory stimuli. If this ability is impaired, there is an altered state of consciousness. Impairment can occur in the sense of impaired level of consciousness, content of consciousness or both [4].

Confusion affects the content of consciousness, and the patient thus has a disorder of attention and concentration, temporal-spatial orientation, memory and/or perception (does not recognise certain places, people, names, etc.). The confused patient is not coherent in thought and actions. Confusion is a syndrome and not a disease, and the aetiology of confusional syndromes is varied [4].

Neurological focal lesions can also cause a confusional syndrome. Examples are subdural haematomas, strokes, brain tumours, encephalitis and meningitis. Delirium is a specific confusional syndrome with varied cognitive and behavioural symptoms, with acute onset (onset within hours or days), characterised by disturbance of attention and perception, with visual hallucinations, agitation, vegetative disturbances and fluctuations in symptom intensity (worsening in the evening) [4].

Akinetic mutism occurs through bifrontal lesions or hydrocephalus and is characterised by the preservation of consciousness, with the inability to initiate voluntary movements and verbal expression, even under nociceptive stimulation. It should be distinguished not only from comatose states but also from psychogenic conditions, periodic paralysis, Guillain-Barré syndrome (GBS) or myasthenia gravis [4].

In the clinical assessment of coma, the practitioner needs to determine whether or not neurological signs of outbreak are present and whether the patient has meningeal syndrome. In this way, he obtains important information about the neurological or toxic-metabolic aetiology of the coma [4].

LP is indicated in all cases where meningitis is suspected and in all patients with suspected SAH in whom CT screening is negative [3].

2.1.3 Fever

Symptoms of meningitis include fever along with other specific symptoms.

2.1.4 Sensitivity to light (photophobia)

Light sensitivity (photophobia) occurs in both meningitis and SAH symptoms.

2.1.5 Seizures

Seizures are quite common and the causes are extremely diverse (multiple sclerosis, meningitis, SAH, etc.).

Advances in the understanding of seizure types and the use of new types of antiepileptic drugs (AEDs) have increased the ability of the emergency physician to accurately diagnose the cause of a patient's seizures and to rationally and systematically treat both the underlying abnormality and the seizures it produces [3].

LP is done when a CNS infection is suspected, and there are no signs of increased intracranial pressure. The pressure at the opening is recorded, and CSF is collected for blood counts including leukocyte count (WBC), protein, glucose, Gram stain, acid-fast bacilli (Ziehl-Neelsen), cryptococcal antigen, Venereal Disease Research Laboratory (VDRL) test, bacterial culture and counterimmunoelectrophoresis or agglutination reactions for bacterial antigens. It is important to note that CSF tests may indicate pleocytosis after a single simple or complex partial seizure, a generalised tonic-clonic seizure or status epilepticus (SE). If a CNS infection is suspected, its treatment is not delayed on the assumption that pleocytosis is due to seizures alone [3].

2.1.6 Gait disorders

Gait disorders are a common finding in the emergency department and usually reflect a nervous system disorder. Orthostasis and gait are unique to each person and reflect gender, age, body habitus, mood and even culture. The purpose of the assessment is to determine the part(s) of the nervous system involved in the type of gait observed [3].

Normal pressure hydrocephalus, a CSF circulation disorder, typically begins with progressive gait difficulties, which are the most marked symptom of the disease [5].

Steps are very small and hesitant, and the feet tend to be "drawn", as if "magnetised", to the floor. Patients may be slightly off-balance towards the back [3].

2.1.7 Dizziness

The word dizziness is a non-specific term used by both patients and medical professionals to describe a disturbance in sensation of well-being; dizziness is usually perceived as altered spatial orientation. Vertigo is defined as the illusion of movement of one's own body or surroundings. Dizziness or vertigo can be the result of numerous disorders of the complex human balance system. Despite the inherent complexity, the assessment of dizziness or vertigo in the emergency department can be simplified by adopting a systematic approach to the history, somatic examination and laboratory investigations. A useful diagnostic method is to determine whether the patient's symptoms are due to disturbance of the vestibular or non-vestibular systems [3].

The central causes of these complaints are generally cerebrovascular disorders, infections (meningitis and encephalitis) and demyelinating diseases.

Traumatised patients with suspected stroke or meningitis will undergo the necessary examinations: CT, MRI or CSF examination, with as little mobilisation as possible and under antiemetic-antivertigo medication. These investigations may be postponed in other situations such as multiple sclerosis, relapsing vertigo without alarming neuronal signs, etc. [6].

2.1.8 Decreased muscle strength ("muscle weakness")

Decreased muscle strength (muscle weakness or muscle strength deficiency) is a condition where the muscles can no longer exert normal force. The inability to perform a specific normal activity suggests decreased muscle strength, which can easily be differentiated from decreased energy or endurance [3].

Decreased muscle strength implies an inability to perform usual activities due to decreased muscle, nerve or upper motor neuron function, not decreased energy or endurance (stamina) [3].

Acute inflammatory demyelinating polyneuropathy, also known as GBS, is the most common nerve root injury to reach emergency departments. The criteria required for the clinical diagnosis of GBS are decreased muscle strength with fairly symmetrical distribution and hypo- or areflexia [3].

In the initial phase, in the presence of numbness and decreased muscle strength with ascending character, a high index of suspicion of GBS is necessary, as auxiliary investigations may not be of any help. Normal CSF protein levels in the initial phase or the finding of numerous lymphocytes do not exclude the diagnosis of GBS. Towards the end of the first week of illness, CSF examination usually shows normal CSF pressure and elevated protein but without leucocytosis, which is called albumin-cytological dissociation [3].

2.2 Representative clinical aspects for which CSF analysis is essential

CSF examination is an essential tool in the diagnosis of certain neurological diseases. It aims to establish appearance, chemical and cytological composition and CSF pressure.

- the appearance of the fluid (under normal conditions, the fluid is clear and perfectly transparent);
- cytological study (normal CSF contains 1-5 figurative elements/mm^3, mainly lymphocytes);
- chemical composition study (normal cerebrospinal fluid proteins are 20-35 mg/dl; normal glycoprotein is 60 mg/dl);
- CSF pressure (normal CSF pressure is 65-195 mmH2O or 15 mm Hg).

2.2.1 Benign intracranial hypertension

Synonyms—Pseudotumor cerebri, idiopathic intracranial hypertension.

Definition—Benign intracranial hypertension is a syndrome of increased intracranial pressure that occurs in the absence of an intracranial tumour or hydrocephalus. Synonyms pseudotumor cerebri or idiopathic intracranial hypertension is preferred because the course of this morbid entity is not always benign. Although rarely life-threatening, increased intracranial pressure may result in permanent loss of vision due to optic nerve damage [1].

Pathophysiology

1. The underlying cause of the elevated intracranial pressure is not known, but it is thought to result from a mismatch between spinal fluid production and absorption or increased resistance to absorption or functional lateral venous sinus obstruction.
2. Traction from swelling or pressure of dilated venous sinuses on pain-sensitive, large cerebral vessels may produce headache.
3. Obesity, anaemia and use of substances such as oestrogen-containing contraceptives, vitamin A or tetracycline may affect spinal fluid balance and provoke the condition [7].

Signs and symptoms—Almost all patients present with generalised headache, daily or almost daily, of fluctuating intensity, sometimes associated with nausea. They may have transient visual impairment, diplopia (due to dysfunction of cranial nerve pair VI) and intracranial, pulsatile tinnitus. Vision loss begins peripherally and may not be noticed by the patient until late in the course of the disease. The main danger is permanent loss of vision [8].

Bilateral papilledema is almost always present. There are a few patients who are asymptomatic but have palpebral oedema discovered on routine ophthalmoscopic examination. Neurological examination may reveal partial cranial VI nerve paresis which otherwise goes unnoticed [8].

The diagnosis is clinically suspected and is confirmed by brain imaging tests (preferably MRI with magnetic resonance venography) and by LP in which increased pressure with normal CSF composition occurs [8].

Treatment

1. Medical therapy is used for patients without visual loss and includes

    a. A medication, usually acetazolamide, to lower intracranial pressure

    b. Weight loss, if appropriate

    c. Steroids are used by some clinicians if visual loss is present.

2. Surgical therapy is reserved for patients with visual loss or poor response to medical therapy and includes

    a. Cerebrospinal fluid (CSF) shunting procedures, especially lumboperitoneal shunt

    b. Optic nerve sheath fenestration, which some believe to be the best procedure to preserve vision

    c. Stenting of functional lateral venous sinus obstruction is under study [7].

2.2.2 Intracranial hypertension (ICH)

The intact skull and spine, together with the relatively inelastic dura, make up a rigid structure (like a container), so increasing the volume of any of its components—brain, blood or CSF—will increase intracranial pressure [5].

ICH is caused by many things: intracranial expansive processes, stroke, infections (meningitis, encephalitis), cerebral oedema, hydrocephalus, CSF accumulation in the cranial cavity and hypertension in the cerebral vessels.

Clinical manifestations of ICH in children and adults are headache, nausea and vomiting, drowsiness, eye paresis and papillary oedema [5].

2.2.3 Intracranial hypotension

Pathogenic mechanisms involved in the occurrence of the condition:

- CSF loss;

- reduced CSF production.

Clinical picture: migraine in orthostatic position (as postpunctional migraine), mild meningismus; rare: cranial nerve deficits (abducens nerve), nausea, vomiting, unsystematised vertigo, tinnitus (possibly due to intralabyrinthine pressure change) [9].

Additional diagnosis

- CSF examination
- CSF pressure < 6 cm H2O (similar to “blind puncture”, air is sucked into the subarachnoid space), CSF must be aspirated with syringe
- slight pleocytosis (lymphocytic) (possible by meningeal irritation), slight protein increase (possible by reduced CSF flow into lumbar subarachnoid space)
- cytology: differential diagnosis with neoplastic meningitis [9]

2.2.4 Hydrocephalus

The term “hydrocephalus” means “water in the head” in Greek.

Hydrocephalus can be due to broadly two mechanisms that can be grouped into two categories: (1) excessive CSF production and (2) decreased CSF reabsorption, which may be caused by a mechanical obstruction located anywhere in the ventricular and cisternal CSF pathways, or by a reabsorption defect itself [10].

In adults, the most common causes are degenerative brain diseases, tumours, strokes, infections and haemorrhages.

Normal pressure hydrocephalus (NPH) is a syndrome that occurs in the elderly and consists of dementia, gait disorder and urinary incontinence associated with ventriculomegaly and normal CSF pressure [3].

Gait disturbance is usually the first symptom of NPH, an important clinical element that differentiates NPH from other dementias. Also, the severity of gait disturbance is the best predictor of clinical improvement following ventriculo-peritoneal shunting. Gait abnormalities are characterised by the widened base of support, hesitant gait onset (apraxia) and frequent falls [3].

LP, rarely indicated by the emergency department in the absence of suspicion of other pathological processes, shows CSF pressure values of 80 to 150 mm water column (H_2O) and normal CSF analysis. Some patients with NPH have temporary improvements in gait disturbance and cognitive functioning after extraction of 20-50 ml of CSF (spinal tap test) [3].

2.2.5 Subarachnoid haemorrhage (SAH)

SAH is a non-traumatic cerebral haemorrhage in which blood extravasates into the meningeal spaces at the subarachnoid level (between the arachnoid and pia mater). The most common cause of SAH is ruptured aneurysms in the pial vessels (more than 80% of cases). Rarer causes are cerebral arteriovenous malformations (AVMs), cavernous malformations, arterial hypertension (AH), arterial dissections, coagulopathies, mycotic aneurysms, brain tumours, dural fistulas [4].

Core Features

1. Thunderclap headache. ‘Worst headache of my life’. Sudden headache that is maximal in intensity at onset is highly suspicious for (SAH) but more gradual headaches are also compatible with this diagnosis. Some patients may have a history of thunderclap headache prior to SAH (‘sentinel bleed’).

2. Altered level of consciousness.The level of arousal at presentation correlates with prognosis. A clear sensorium predicts better outcomes; coma portends the worst prognosis.

3. Non-contrast head CT shows blood in the subarachnoid space. The sensitivity of non-contrast head CT for SAH within hours of bleeding is very high when read by an experienced neuroradiologist. As blood resolves, sensitivity decreases, and only 50% of patients will have subarachnoid blood on non-contrast head CT 1 week following the bleed.

4. Blood and blood products (bilirubin) in the cerebrospinal fluid (CSF). The absence of red blood cells (RBCs) in the CSF at the time of presentation excludes the diagnosis of SAH. Xanthochromia, a yellow tinge of the CSF due to the presence of bilirubin, may not be observable at onset as it develops within 12 hours of bleeding and dissipates within 3 weeks.

5. Cerebral aneurysm visualised on CT or MR angiogram. Conventional catheter cerebral angiography is traditionally considered the gold standard for diagnosis of cerebral aneurysms, but the non-invasive CTA can detect aneurysms as small as 2 mm in diameter and is usually adequate for ruling out aneurysms [11].

2.2.6 Central nervous system (CNS) infections

Infectious diseases affecting the CNS are numerous and heterogeneous, in both pathogenic mechanisms and clinical manifestations. All known types of infectious agents (bacteria, viruses, fungi, parasites, prions) can affect the nervous system, either directly or by triggering a pathological immune response with a cross-mechanism. Certain neuroinfections, such as those with *Treponema pallidum*, *Borrelia burgdorferi*, Koch's bacillus or human immunodeficiency virus, can take many forms and cause almost any neurological sign [4].

From the beginning, it should be noted that the diagnosis of the vast majority of neuroinfections requires LP, as CSF is the only CNS biological sample that is relatively easy to access [4].

Clinical manifestations of CNS infections are fever, headache, altered mental status—lethargy and confusion, seizures, neurological signs of outbreak and headache [12].

Depending on the location of the infection and clinical manifestations will be grouped into several major syndromes: encephalitic syndrome, meningeal syndrome and myelitis syndrome [4].

Acute bacterial meningitis

Acute bacterial meningitis is fulminant, with fatal pyogenic infection starting in the meninges. Symptoms include headache, fever and a stiff neck. In the absence of prompt treatment, it progresses to obnubilation and coma. Diagnosis is made by CSF examination [8].

LP with CSF analysis is the essential diagnostic manoeuvre in bacterial meningitis. Characteristic CSF changes are increased pressure, turbulent or purulent macroscopic appearance, pleocytosis (1000-10,000 leukocytes/mm^3), 90% of which are polymorphonuclears, hyperproteinaemia (100-500 mg/dl), low glycoproteinaemia (below 40 mg/dl). In addition, Gram staining of the CSF sediment is performed, which in most cases identifies germs. In addition to blood cultures, it is useful also to seed CSF on culture medium and perform antibiogram. Enzyme-linked immunosorbent assay (ELISA), polymerase chain reaction (PCR) or immunoelectrophoresis are required for aetiological diagnosis of infection [4].

Brain abscess

Brain abscess is an infection located in the brain parenchyma, following spread from a nearby septic focus (otomastoiditis, sinusitis—this is why it frequently occurs in the temporal lobe), remote seeding (in endocarditis, pneumonia, patients with cardiac malformations, even dental infections) or by direct inoculation of germs (TCC or neurosurgical intervention) [4].

It manifests clinically as a space replacement process (headache and nausea/vomiting) associated with febrile syndrome, altered consciousness and focal neurological signs, depending on the location [4].

CSF culture-based inoculation can often identify the pathogen and antibiotics can guide treatment [4].

Subdural empyema

Subdural empyema is a collection of pus located between the dura mater and the arachnoid. Symptoms include fever, lethargy, focal neurological deficits and seizures [8].

Brain CT or preferably brain MRI (which better shows interhemispheric and hemispheric convexity collections) and CSF with high protein numbers, modest pleocytosis (50 leukocytes/mm3), and low glucose clear the diagnosis [4].

Epidural abscess

Epidural ("peridural") abscess is a suppurative collection that may be located in the skull or spinal cord between the dura mater and the inner bony plate of the skull or vertebral arch. Seeding often occurs directly, during neurosurgical manoeuvres and trauma, from the vicinity (paranasal sinuses, middle ear, orbit) and less often by haematogenous seeding [4].

Patients with cerebral epidural abscess frequently associate meningitis, brain abscess and subdural empyema. The germs frequently involved are streptococci and staphylococci. CT with contrast or possibly MRI with contrast detects the collection, CSF may be normal if the abscess has not penetrated the subdural or subarachnoid space [4].

Tuberculous meningitis

The incidence of tuberculosis (TB) is on the rise due to an increase in the number of HIV-infected people, homeless people and immigrants from developing countries [3].

In conditions of clinical suspicion for diagnosis, an LP should be performed, preceded by fundoscopic examination, which may identify papillary oedema (common in tuberculous meningitis), optic atrophy or even retinal tuberculosis [4].

CSF typically shows a much-increased proteinaemia (the most important of all meningitis), up to 1000 mg/dl, with fibrin deposits and the sign of the present veil (heating the CSF tube with flame leads to the precipitation of excess proteins and their appearance as a whitish "veil"), low glucose, pleocytosis 100–500 leukocytes/mm^3, of which more than 50% neutrophils. Pleocytosis is usually absent in HIV-positive and immunosuppressed patients. CSF pressure is usually increased. However, the macroscopic appearance is clear, which has led to the classic classification of tuberculous meningitis as "aseptic" meningitis (with clear, non-purulent CSF; aseptic meningitis also includes viral meningitis, carcinomatous meningitis, Lyme meningitis and meningitis from vasculitis and granulomatous diseases). CSF is generally paucibacillary, Koch's bacilli being difficult to detect. Cultures are made by seeding on a special medium (Lowenstein) and then Ziehl-Nielson staining, but slightly more than half of cases can be etiologically diagnosed in this way. The PCR method is much more sensitive but more expensive [4].

Neurosyphilis

Syphilis is a sexually transmitted disease, and the pathogen responsible is *Treponema pallidum*, a Gram-negative spirochete (the spirochete family also includes the *Borrelia* and *Leptospira* genera) [4].

In the CNS, the infection causes chronic inflammation of the meninges, which over time can be complicated by parenchymal lesions [4].

More specific laboratory tests, such as the CSF Venereal Disease Laboratory (VDRL) test or the fluorescence treponemal antibody-antibody absorption test (FTA-ABS), combined with non-specific parameters (CSF pleocytosis greater than nine leukocytes per microscopic visual field of high magnitude, elevated CSF proteins and low glucose levels) are needed for accurate diagnosis of present or antecedent neurosyphilis in the context of the history and physical examination. Except in cases where CSF is contaminated with seropositive blood during lumbar puncture, positive VDRL reaction in CSF indicates previous or current neurosyphilis [3].

Neuroborreliosis

Borreliosis (Lyme disease—borreliosis was named Lyme disease because it was first described in the town of Old Lyme in Connecticut, USA, in 1975) recognises the spirochete *Borrelia burgdorferi* as the infectious agent, which is transmitted to humans through the bite of a tick (*Ixodes ricinus*) [4].

Diagnosis is based on the clinical picture, the presence of lymphocytic meningitis and serological confirmation of infection in serum and CSF. The first method used is usually ELISA (enzyme-linked immunosorbent assay), and in the case of a high titre of anti-*Borrelia* antibodies, Western blot (qualitative and semi-quantitative method of protein identification based on immunological principles) or PCR (polymerase chain reaction) is used for confirmation [4].

Encephalitis

Encephalitis is inflammation of the brain parenchyma due to direct viral invasion or hypersensitivity triggered by a virus or other foreign protein. Encephalomyelitis is the same process but involves the brain and spinal cord. These conditions can be caused by a variety of viruses. Symptoms consist of fever, headache and altered consciousness, often associated with seizures or focal neurological deficits. Diagnosis requires CSF analysis and neuroimaging investigations [8].

The diagnosis of encephalitis is suspected in patients with unexplained alterations in consciousness. If encephalitis is present, CSF analysis shows lymphocytic pleocytosis, normal glucose, slightly increased proteinaemia and absence of pathogens on culture and Gram stain (similar appearance to aseptic meningitis); CSF changes may occur 8-24 hours after the onset of symptoms. In case of haemorrhagic necrosis, CSF will show a lot of red blood cells and few neutrophils, increasing proteinuria and glycoradiation moderately decreasing. PCR analysis in CSF to identify herpes virus is sensitive and specific, but obtaining results may take time. Viral CSF cultures may show growth of enterovirus but less of other viruses. CSF and blood tests in both the acute and convalescent phases should be spaced a few weeks apart as they may show an increase in viral titre specific to certain viral infections [8].

Neurocysticercosis

Neurocysticercosis is the most common brain parasitosis and occurs following ingestion of pork infested with *Taenia solium* eggs. When they occur, the clinical manifestations consist of epileptic seizures, generalised or partial, migraine-type headache and behavioural disorders (Garg, 1988) [4].

Diagnosis involves evidence of cysticerci and perilesional oedema by brain CT or MRI (round, small, hypodense images on CT and hypointense in T1 sequence on MRI, possibly with calcifications), CSF with mononuclear pleocytosis, hyperproteinaemia, normal glucose, elevated IgG and sometimes oligoclonal bands, leucocytosis, with eosinophilia and ELISA with elevated CSF antibody titres [4].

Creutzfeldt-Jakob disease

Creutzfeldt-Jacob disease is a sporadic or familial prion disease. Bovine spongiform encephalopathy (mad cow disease) is a variant of the disease. Symptoms include dementia, myoclonus and other neurological deficits, with death occurring within 1-2 years [8].

CSF is biochemically and cellularly normal but contains elevated levels of 14-3-3 protein (assay has sensitivity and specificity over 90%) [4].

2.2.7 Demyelinating diseases

Multiple sclerosis

Multiple sclerosis (MS) is the most common form of demyelinating disease of the nervous system, with an autoimmune mechanism—i.e. abnormal production of antibodies directed against the destruction of the body's own tissues/cells [12].

MS is characterised by areas of demyelination, spread throughout the brain and spinal cord. Common symptoms of MS are visual and oculomotor abnormalities, paraesthesia, muscle weakness, spasticity, urinary dysfunction and mild cognitive impairment [8].

CSF examination is altered in over 90% of patients. Moderate monocytic pleocytosis (dozens of cells/mm^3) occurs mostly at onset and during episodes, corresponding to an exacerbation of the inflammatory process. In about half of patients, proteinaemia is above normal limits. The appearance of oligoclonal bands in the CSF (expression of immunoglobulins synthesised in the nervous system) is a test with high sensitivity (more than 90% of patients) but low specificity. In the same situation is the immunoglobulin index, which is calculated according to the formula: (CSF IgG/serum IgG): (CSF albumin/serum albumin), whose value greater than 1.7 is suggestive of diagnosis (normal value is around 1) [4].

2.2.8 Peripheral neuropathies

Guillain-Barré syndrome (GBS)

GBS (Acute idiopathic polyneuritis, Landry's palsy, acute inflammatory demyelinating polyneuropathy) is a rapidly progressive inflammatory polyneuropathy characterised by muscle weakness and mild loss of distal sensation. The cause appears to be autoimmune. Diagnosis is clinical and treatment consists of plasmapheresis, administration of gamma globulin and, in severe cases, mechanical ventilation [8].

GBS can occur at any age. About 5-7 days after the onset of motor deficit, PL shows typical (pathognomonic) CSF biochemical changes: increased proteinaemia without pleocytosis (albumin-cytokine dissociation) [4].

3. Conclusions

Therefore, in addition to clinical aspects, CSF analysis is extremely useful in the diagnosis of certain neurological disorders.

Conflict of interest

The author declare no conflict of interest.

Abbreviations

CSF	cerebrospinal fluid
LP	lumbar puncture
CNS	central nervous system
ICH	intracranial hypertension
CT	computer tomography
SAH	subarachnoid haemorrhage
TBI	traumatic brain injury
GBS	Guillain-Barré syndrome
AEDS	antiepileptic drugs
SE	status epilepticus
NPH	normal pressure hydrocephalus
CNS	central nervous system
MS	multiple sclerosis

Author details

Mariana-Alis Neagoe[1,2]

1 “Titu Maiorescu” University, Faculty of Medicine, Bucharest, Romania

2 Memormed Medical Centre, Bucharest, Romania

*Address all correspondence to: dr.alisneagoe2011@yahoo.com

References

[1] Weatherall DJ, Ledingham JGG, Warrell DA. Treatise on Neurology Medicine. Bucharest: Editura Tehnică; 2000. p. 41, 256, 273

[2] Băjenaru O. Diagnostic and Treatment Guidelines in Neurology. Bucharest: Editura Medicală Amaltea; 2005. p. 153

[3] Shah SM, Kelly KM. Principles and Practice of Emergency Neurology. Bucharest: Medicală; 2012. p. 51, 58, 61, 63-64, 73, 77-78, 81, 107, 120, 129-130, 141-142, 144, 212, 306-307

[4] Bogdan OP, Ovidiu B. Essential Elements in Clinical Neurology. Bucharest: Editura Medicală Amaltea; 2009. p. 80, 190-191, 204, 208, 212-221, 229, 231-234, 239-240, 243-244

[5] Ropper AH, Samuels MA, Klein JP, editors. Adams and Victor Principles and Practice of Clinical Neurology. 10th ed. Bucharest: Callisto Medical Publishing House; 2017. p. 122, 620-621

[6] Szatmári S, Szász JA. Neurological Emergencies. Târgu Mureş: Farmamedia Publishing House; 2007. p. 75

[7] Martin AS, Allan HR. Samuel's Manual of Neurologic Therapeutics. 19th ed. Philadelphia: Wolters Kluwer; 2017. pp. 432-433

[8] Mark HB, Robert SP. The Merk Manual. 18th ed. Bucharest: ALL Publishing House; 2006. p. 1846, 1851-1853, 1857-1858, 1888, 1894-1895

[9] Hufschmidt A, Lücking CH. Comprehensive Neurology from Symptom to Treatment. Bucharest: Polirom; 2002. p. 207

[10] Tiberiu P. Nuclear Magnetic Resonance in Clinical Diagnosis. Bucharest: Editura Medicală; 1995. p. 221

[11] Ilya K, José B. Top 100 Diagnoses in Neurology Wolters. Philadelphia: Kluwer Publishing House; 2021. p. 230

[12] Robert RM. Neurological Disorders for all, M.A.S.T. Bucharest: Publishing House; 2006. p. 115, 131

Chapter 4

Basic CSF Tests Should Go beyond Early in Atypical Presentations of Brain Infections

Kanwal Altaf Malik, Babu Paturi and Stephane Maingard

Abstract

The spectrum of infections in the central nervous system (CNS) has dramatically changed over centuries, attributing to high rate of microbial replication, mutations, and expansion across the new geographical regions. Vaccination reduced the burden of bacterial meningitis; however, serotype replacement, for example, *S. pneumoniae* remains a problem. Urgent blood and cerebrospinal fluid (CSF) sampling is recommended unless lumbar puncture is contraindicated. CSF Gram stain and culture, serology, and polymerase chain reaction (PCR) are the basic tests in isolating the organism. About 40 to 60% of CNS infections has undetermined diagnosis due to lack of standardised diagnostic tests and clinical case definitions that may lead to inappropriate use of antibiotics or untreated infection with long-term sequelae. Among case examples, Lyme cerebellitis presents with ataxia and nystagmus, with diagnostic delay and resultant delay in treatment. Early inclusion of specific advanced tests on CSF, molecular diagnostics serology, and next-generation sequencing (NGS) involves a comprehensive quantitative analysis of all pathogens. CfDNA has high sensitivity (75–91%) and specificity (81–100%) to detect any intracellular or extracellular pathogens. Early inclusion of CSF basic tests to beyond by including current evidence-based technology tools in conjunction with clinical presentation could improve quality in diagnosing early, any rare brain infections.

Keywords: cerebrospinal fluid infections, meningitis, encephalitis, meningoencephalitis, whole genome sequencing, molecular diagnostic serology

1. Introduction

The spectrum of infections in central nervous system (CNS) has dramatically changed over centuries, attributing to high rate of microbial replication, mutations, and expansion across the new geographic regions [1–13]. During the later twentieth century there has been a dramatic change in CNS infections. In 1950, with introduction of penicillin, neurosyphilis was eradicated, while mass vaccination eradicated poliomyelitis. The vaccines against microbes, like *Streptococcus pneumoniae*, *Neisseria meningitidis*, *Haemophilus influenzae* type B (Hib) has reduced the burden of bacterial meningitis [1, 2]. However, the serotype replacement of *S. pneumoniae* with decreased sensitivity to antibiotics, and other microbes including neurotropic arbovirus, enteroviruses have continued to raised concerns [2–4].

Central nervous system (CNS) infections, including meningitis, encephalitis, and meningoencephalitis, are caused by a variety of pathogens, primarily viruses and bacteria. Parasites and fungus are less common. Some infectious agents, such as enteroviruses (EVs), commonly causes meningitis, while others, like herpes simplex virus-1 (HSV-1), primarily causes encephalitis. For a definite microbiological diagnosis, many complementary diagnostic tests should be selected, often performed parallel, that varies case-by-case, within the clinical context. Around 40 to 60% of CNS infections remains undiagnosed, due to absence of clinical case definitions and standardised diagnostic tests, leading to inappropriate use of antibiotics and incompletely treated infection with long term morbidity and sequelae [5–8]. Constellation of clinical findings, CSF investigation and neuroimaging may be crucial for diagnosis. Epidemiological factors can further help any other investigations. The clinical guidelines recommend urgent blood and CSF sampling unless lumbar puncture is contraindicated due to raised intracranial pressure. An ideal diagnostic test should detect early all possible infectious agents, and a high negative predictive value, to rule out any infection rapidly, with minimal laboratory work. However, there is no such ideal test and limitations remain in rapid diagnosis of CNS infections [14].

2. Diagnostic challenges and case reports

Acute bacterial meningitis, encephalitis, or meningoencephalitis is a medical emergency. Typical presentation of meningitis which is inflammation of meninges, includes fever, headache, and neck stiffness, so diagnosis is relatively easy. However, meningitis may cause adjacent brain parenchyma inflammation, called as meningoencephalitis. It may lack the classic symptom triad of meningitis with atypical and insidious clinical manifestations including mixed neuropsychiatric symptoms, resulting in diagnostic difficulties and delay in treatment [15]. Encephalitis is interchangeably used with encephalopathy due to clinical overlap, however they may present distinct pathophysiologic process, where encephalopathy is altered mental state or cognitive impairment, with or without inflammation of the brain tissue [8].

2.1 Case 1

2.1.1 Group B Streptococcus in adult presenting with mania

A case is reported in a 74-year-old woman with GBS meningoencephalitis. She presented with shortness of breath, cough, and chest pain after a month of successfully treated COVID 19 upper respiratory tract infection with monoclonal antibody treatment. She had medical and psychiatric comorbidities including diabetes mellitus, hypertension, hyperlipidaemia, obesity, fatty liver disease, anxiety disorder, and splenectomy. On presentation, she required some oxygen support consistent with her chest findings, while her neurological exam was normal. However, later she developed newly onset paranoid psychosis, and distrustful behaviour towards staff and visitors. The main symptom in the patient was mania that continued to worsen, without any classic symptoms of fever, neck stiffness and headache. On investigations, she had raised inflammatory markers that continued to rise despite of antibiotics (cefepime, doxycycline, levofloxacin), blood culture showed no growth. Among relevant neurological investigations, CT brain was normal and CSF analysis showed no growth on culture, however the PCR detected *Streptococcus agalactiae*. She was treated with intravenous ceftriaxone and lithium. She fully recovered and her behaviour returned to baseline [16].

2.1.2 Discussion

Streptococcus agalactiae, also known as group B Streptococcus (GBS), is a common pathogen in the neonatal period that can cause meningitis and sepsis. This is a rare cause of meningitis in non-pregnant adults. This case illustrates an unusual presentation of a new infection in elderly with *streptococcus agalactiae* with mania as a predominant symptom, a very rarely reported presenting manifestation of acute bacterial meningitis. A patient who is already on broad spectrum antibiotics, diagnosing CSF infection can be challenging with CSF culture, as in this case where the culture showed no growth. However, PCR assays may increase the diagnostic accuracy of CSF with high sensitivity and specificity, despite on treatment [16, 17].

2.2 Case 2

2.2.1 Late onset HSV encephalitis

A 22-day old baby girl presented to the emergency department with a history of fever and associated jerky movements of left upper limb each lasting for about 5 secs, continuing every 2 to 3 hrs. Her initial examination at presentation to ER was normal, including neurological exam. Baseline investigations were normal. CSF analysis showed elevated white cell count 98 and RBC 0. CSF culture was negative. Baby was started empirically on cefotaxime and acyclovir. It was uneventful pregnancy, with no history of herpetic lesions in mother and no perinatal or post-natal abnormalities [18]. Her initial CSF PCR came positive for HSV1. MRI showed infarction of the right internal capsule to the vertex. EEG demonstrated asymmetry in the frontal-central location. She was treated with acyclovir IV for 21 days followed by acyclovir PO for 6 months. She was followed by paediatric team and physiotherapy. She continued to have left sided hemiparesis on the left upper limb which was improved gradually with minimal residual weakness [19].

2.2.2 Discussion

This case presents a mild presentation in form of temperature and some jerky movements,but not overt seizures with associated deterioration. However, a high index of suspicion and early empirical management was crucial before any final diagnosis. A combination of CSF PCR, MRI and EEG led to the final diagnosis of HSV encephalitis. Despite of early empirical treatment, there was a residual morbidity. On the contrary, in the absence of any antiviral therapy mortality is reported as 40–50% [20].

2.3 Case 3

2.3.1 Lyme cerebellar encephalomyelitis presenting with ocular signs

A 5-year-old boy presented with newly onset funny turns of head towards left side and 'shaky' eyes. Preceding history of pyrexia and night sweats for 5 days. On examination, he had horizontal and torsional nystagmus with left lateral gaze, compensatory head tilt towards left side, and gait ataxia. He later developed fever, neck pain, lethargy, and headache [21, 22]. Inflammatory markers were unremarkable, Mantoux test was negative. MRI brain had T2/FLAIR with high signal in the left hemisphere of cerebellum. CSF analysis after lumbar puncture showed elevated WCC of 579 mm3 (79%lymph), and a low glucose of 2.3 mmol/L. CSF culture showed no growth and PCRs were negative for viruses and bacteria including HSV1, HSV2, CMV, VZV, Para echovirus, enterovirus, pneumococcus, meningococcal, and haemophilus influenza respectively. Extended viral panel nasal swab was negative. Empirically he was treated with IV acyclovir (4 days) and cefotaxime (10 days) and rationalised based on results from CSF. He had residual nystagmus on extreme left lateral gaze, however significant improvement was observed. Subsequent blood tests were positive for *Borrelia Burgdorferi* immunoblot and enzyme immunoassay. *B. Burgdorferi* IgG/IgM (C6 EIA) was highly positive highlighting recent/current Lyme disease. The IgM immunoblot was strongly positive to borrelia antigens P41, Osp17 and OspC, while IgG immunoblot was strongly positive to borrelia antigens P14 and V1se antigens. There was no history of tick bite or any recent travel, however the patient parents had a forest in their land, located in a rural area of west of Ireland. After consultation with infectious disease, he was managed as Lyme disease and received outpatient antibiotic treatment with ceftriaxone 1.75 g OD for 21 days [9, 23].

2.3.2 *Discussion*

This case with CNS Lyme disease was a diagnostic challenge. Lyme encephalomyelitis is rare in Lyme neuroborreliosis, presenting with facial nerve palsies and meningitis. The basic CSF tests, however, were not diagnostic with insufficient evidence on history leading to a delay in diagnosis. Any advance CSF analysis on the contrary would have picked the diagnosis of Lyme encephalomyelitis early, leading to early management.

2.4 Case 4

2.4.1 *Fatal pneumococcal meningitis in a vaccinated child*

A 2 year and 4 months old boy presented with febrile seizure, glasgow coma scale (GCS) 4/15, and unequal pupils on examination. He had a fever, productive cough, vomiting and decreased oral intake for 2 days. At 04.30 hrs parents saw him moaning. At 08.30 hrs he was limp followed by high temperature of 40 C and seizures at 10.08 hrs. On arrival to ED, he was intubated due to prolonged seizures and low GCS. Fluid bolus was given followed by septic workup and empirical treatment with IV ceftriaxone and acyclovir. He had history of asthma, recurrent lower respiratory tract infection, and febrile seizure in past. He was developmentally appropriate for age and vaccinated up to date including Pneumococcal conjugate vaccine (PCV13). Blood tests revealed high white cell count, neutrophilia, and significantly raised CRP. CXR was consistent with left lower lobe and right hilum consolidation with bilateral perihilar thickening of bronchial walls. CT brain showed signs of significantly raised intracranial pressure and cerebral oedema due to global hypoxic event. IV Mannitol, Dexamethasone, and Vancomycin were added while the child remained intubated. Later blood culture turned out positive for *Streptococcus pneumoniae*, and blood PCR isolated Serotype 24 B on sub typing. MRI brain on the following day showed cerebral oedema with tonsillar herniation. The child was declared dead the same day.

2.4.2 *Discussion*

Streptococcus pneumoniae is the most common cause of bacterial meningitis in infants. It remains an important cause of morbidity and mortality in children. Despite of immunisation, Pneumococcal meningitis may still occur from non-vaccine serotypes, whereby a history of vaccination can distract consideration of pneumococcal infection. As demonstrated in this case, the subtype 24 B resulted in meningitis with a fatal outcome, outside the strains that are used in used in vaccine i.e. PCV13 and other types of vaccine that were used in the past PPV 23, PCV 7, PCV 10.

2.5 Case 5

2.5.1 *Sudden and unexplained neonatal death with Group A Streptococcus infection*

Group A streptococcus (GAS) is a rare infection in neonates. The mode of transmission in most invasive late onset cases is unknown. Vertical transmission or postnatal acquisition of focal GAS infection such as pharyngitis and episiotomy abscess are probable sources of transmission. A term baby, with history of uneventful pregnancy and delivery, presented to emergency with poor feeding and reduced activity. At presentation, on examination he had normal vitals, intermittent grunting, hypotonia, and poor response on stimulation. Septic work up results showed WCC = 1.6, neutrophils = 1.02, lymphocytes = 0.29, platelets were out of range, prolonged PT of 22.8, CRP 186.4, lactate = 4. He was treated with IV antibiotics as per the local antimicrobial protocol. Within 1 hour of presentation, he deteriorated with apnoeic episodes, and poor capillary refill >4 secs. From airway point of view, he got intubated and ventilated, circulation; received 3 IV normal saline 20 ml/kg boluses. He was started on dopamine, nor adrenaline and mannitol was given followed by transfer to a tertiary ICU. His blood culture came positive at 9 hrs for Group A *Streptococcus pyogenes*. Despite of adequate treatment, his condition continued to deteriorate, resulting in eventually withdrawal of care, and declared dead after 12 hours of presentation [24].

2.5.2 *Discussion*

Usually, Group B streptococcus pneumonia is the causative agent of neonatal sepsis, meningitis, however in this case Group A strep unexpectedly caused neonatal sepsis, with suspected meningitis. The outcome was fatal. A high index of suspicion is crucial in a an acutely unwell baby [24].

3. Advances in diagnosing CSF infections from basic to beyond

WHO global initiative to eliminate meningitis from worldwide by 2030 has five pillars of the road map, where one of the pillar is "Diagnosis and treatment", that aim for comprehensive, reliable and cost-effective diagnostic investigations [18].

3.1 Cerebrospinal fluid (CSF) culture

CSF culture is the gold standard test for diagnosing acute bacterial meningitis by detecting viable bacteria from the meninges. However, inflammation of CSF evident by pleocytosis, predominantly neutrophils, high protein levels, and hypoglycorrhachia, is an indirect evidence of acute bacterial meningitis, that leads to empirical management before final CSF culture is reported or in cases when pathogen remains unidentified. CSF culture is 100% specific. The limitations to CSF culture pertain to its sample handling e.g., volume, transport, and storage. The sensitivity varies among different pathogens for e.g., *Neisseria meningitidis* is not detected within 2 hours of initiation of treatment, *S. pneumoniae* is detected up to 8 hours. Also, any prior use of antibiotics may affect viability of bacteria to grow on culture, that reduces the sensitivity of CSF culture. The sensitivity of CSF culture for tuberculous meningitis is 60%, that is increased to >85% by repeated lumbar puncture and multiple samples [4, 21].

3.2 Point of care assay

Point of care assays include latex agglutination and lateral flow assay. Sero-agglutination assays depends on the expression of polysaccharide capsule as target antigen. Cross-reactivity prevents characterisation of definite isolate due to poly-agglutination. Lateral flow assays, make use of antibodies, for e.g. Meningo Speed rapid diagnostic, immunochromatographic test that detects meningococcal serogroups in CSF. Others include, Nucleic acid lateral flow immunoassay, that detects antigen-antibody interaction, Nucleic acid lateral flow assay, that detects specific hybridised nucleic acid amplicons. They are fast, cheap, and easy test, however limited by its clinical relevance if done solely and their susceptibility to bacterial viability [22].

3.3 Molecular tool assay

Molecular tools for CSF analysis are widely popular, they include polymerase chain reaction (PCR), quantitative or qualitative (qPCR), real-time PCR (rtPCR), and loop-mediated isothermal amplification assays (LAMP). Molecular assays are more specific and sensitive than culture. Studies have shown that 30–50% of negative culture will have positive PCR, that challenge the traditional gold standard investigations for diagnosing acute bacterial meningitis. However, this raises a concern where PCR is not widely available and the diagnosis is solely dependent on CSF culture, if the patient treatment given is suboptimal in terms of dose and course of antibiotics. The use of prior antibiotics before CSF testing affects the yield of microbes on CSF culture, while PCR can still be positive, demonstrates its clinical relevance and utility. PCR detects a single pathogen, and multiplex PCR assays detects multiple pathogens reducing time and costs [22]. The specificity of single PCR assays and clinical relevance may be questionable in situations where herpes viruses are positive or in the absence of CSF pleocytosis, it gets challenging to interpret a positive PCR within the clinical context. On animal models, it has been undetermined, as to how early as little as 12 hrs or how long PCR can still be positive in CSF infections. In patients with nasopharyngeal carriage of pneumococcus, there are high rates of false positive CSF PCR [21]. HSV PCR can be falsely negative in children early in the course, suggesting repeat LP within 3–7 days, if the first LP was negative with persistent suspicion on neuroimaging i.e. temporal lobe involvement, along with intrathecal HSV antibodies [20].

World Health Organisation (WHO) recommends rt. PCR for testing meningococcus, pneumococcus, and Hib for suspected meningitis. The challenge in molecular assays remains in their availability especially in developing countries due to limited resources [22].

LAMP works in isothermal condition and amplifies a specific target DNA using a DNA polymerase. It has high specificity. The LAMP assay for Hib discriminates it from other strains of encapsulated *H. influenzae* strains and has more sensitivity than bexA PCR [22].

The single plex rtPCR assays have sensitivities and specificities reported as 91 to 100%. Multiplex assays reported to have sensitivities 73–94% including targeting *N. meningitidis*, *S. pneumoniae*, and *H. influenzae* and high specificities from 98 to 100%. The sensitivity of multiples assays is more than single plex, however specificity is comparable. LAMP assays have high sensitivity 80–100% and specificity 99–100% as compared to rtPCR. LAMP on non-CSF sample i.e. blood and nasopharyngeal samples will have less sensitivity and specificity less then CSF samples, however in invasive meningococcal disease LAMP assays for ctRA have similar sensitivity and specificity for all CSF and non CSF samples [22].

Multiplex PCR assay detects a set of pathogens, predetermined that is highly related to CNS infection. The BioFire FilmArray (FA-MEP) panel is a multiplex PCR, to detect community acquired CNS infection. It tests *Haemophilus influenzae*, *N. meningitidis*, *L. monocytogenes*, *Streptococcus agalactiae*, *S. pneumoniae* and *Escherichia coli*, in viruses VZV, HSV-1, CMV, HSV-2, enterovirus, par echovirus, and HHV-6, and) and fungus *C. neoformans*. It is easy to use and rapid turnaround time. In one of the study FA-MEP had 69.5% of positive samples, with 68% false-positive rate for bacteria predominant *S. pneumoniae* and 22% false positive for viruses. It had low false negatives especially with HHV6, enterovirus, and *S. agalactiae*. Negative predictive value was >99.9% while positive predictive value was 92.5% [14, 25]. The clinical significance is unknown of detecting multiple potential pathogens in one sample and needs further confirmation by microbe specific tests.

3.4 Next generation sequencing

It is a non-culture method that directly detects the genomes of the pathogen in the clinical specimen. It analyses multiple genetic targets directly from genomes.

A review, on studies making use of Next-generation sequencing (NGS), potential pathogens were detected in 22.1% paediatric patients through NGS on CSF. Subsequently confirmed by serologic assays and CSF culture in 6 studies. In 18 out of 26 studies, unknown or unidentified organisms were detected [13]. In one cohort study, the efficiency of cell free DNA (cf DNA) metagenomic NGS in CNS infection and accuracy between cf. DNA and wc DNA (whole cell DNA) was studied. It was found that cfDNA mNGS detected 71% pathogens that correlated with the clinical diagnosis in 67.5%. cfDNA mNGS had more efficacy than wcDNA mNGS for detecting mycobacterium and viruses. The best time for the mNGS ranged from 1 to 6 days after antimicrobials were started and the earlier mNGS used, the better was the detection rate. It demonstrates the superiority of cfDNA mNGS to conventional methods in detecting pathogens in CNS infections.

Next generation sequencing is rapid, diagnostic in patients who are on treatment with rituximab, have high sensitivity independent of specific pathogen primers. Detects microbes in immunocompromised patients, novel viruses, and gives information about molecular epidemiology. It has limitations as it relies on nucleic acid to be present hence it does not detect the immune antibody mediated process. Dependant on replication time, hence viruses with shorter replication are not picked up however in immunocompromised when it has prolonged replication, it can be easily detected. High sensitivity picks up normal commensal in skin. This warrants the use of negative controls to determine the specificity. The clinical application depends on careful consideration of the clinical context and confirming the susceptible microbes with standard testing.

Currently being used as the last resort where, the diagnosis remains unclear. However, it is promising in terms of early detection, without extensive workup and early recognition to optimise management early. Oxford Nanopore sequencing, recently used in Zambia as rapid diagnostic technology for bacterial meningitis sequencing of the 16S rRNA [26]. The limitations are the technical, and financial challenges.

3.5 Neuroimaging

In neuroimaging Magnetic resonance imaging (MRI) is more sensitive and specific as compared to computed tomography (CT), to spot any early changes and exclude alternative diagnosis. MRI, specific findings may relate to certain aetiological microbe like arboviruses or HSV but may not always be helpful to differentiate. Electroencephalogram (EEG) is recommended to exclude non-infectious causes, with non-specific symptoms of altered behaviour [3].

Microbiology (CSF culture)	
Advantages	**Limitations**
Cheap	Prior antibiotics use affect cultivable bacteria
Isolate archived for use in future	Some microbes are difficult to culture
	Time dependant for results
	Specimen quantity, storage and transport can affect the result
Point of care Assay (Lateral flow, Latex agglutination)	
Advantages	**Limitations**
Cheap and easy	Subjective
Rapid	Sensitive to prior antibiotics
	Latex agglutination depends on expression of antigen.
	Cross reactivity
Molecular Assay (PCR and Gel electrophoresis)	
Advantages	**Limitations**
Rapid	Availability
Independent of microbe viability	Multiplex PCR unknown relevance for fungal and bacterial
Multiplex PCR detects multiple predetermined microbes	
Next generation sequencing	
Advantages	**Limitations**
Rapid	Do not detect immune response
Detects easily in immunocompromised	Do not detect viruses with shorter replication time
Detects microbes in patients on rituximab with unreliable antibody	Can detect normal commensal/laboratory reagent due to high sensitivity
Detects novel pathogens	

Table 1.
Advantages and limitations of CSF investigations.

4. Conclusion

The most promising advances in diagnosing CSF infections involve the advanced molecular assays with comparative genomic analyses to improve sensitivity and specificity, to detect alternate diagnostic targets for species-specificity. Availability of databases to store and analyse genomes for comparison e.g. PubMLST databases and BMGAP that store a variety of genomes in dedicated libraries for secure online portal [27, 28]. The role of NGS is more prominent in immunocompromised individuals who are likely more susceptible then than immunocompetent, with insidious course of illness and in those with no clinical improvement despite of empirical treatment with CSF findings suggestive of CNS infection. The ideal diagnostic assay should timely diagnose, and one that detects multiple pathogens at low cost (**Table 1**) [13, 22].

Author details

Kanwal Altaf Malik[1]*, Babu Paturi[2] and Stephane Maingard[3]

1 Royal Belfast Hospital for Sick Children, Belfast Trust, Northern Ireland, UK

2 RCSI Hospital Group, Dublin, Ireland

3 RCSI Our Lady of Lourdes Hospital Drogheda, Ireland

*Address all correspondence to: dr.kanwal.altaf@gmail.com

References

[1] van Ettekoven CN, van de Beek D, Brouwer MC. Update on community-acquired bacterial meningitis: Guidance and challenges. Clinical Microbiology and Infection. 2017;**23**(9):601-606

[2] McIntyre PB, O'Brien KL, Greenwood B, van de Beek D. Effect of vaccines on bacterial meningitis worldwide. Lancet. 2012;**380**(9854): 1703-1711

[3] Paturi B. Fatal Pneumococcal Meningitis in a vaccinated child ESPID-2018-Abstractspdf. 2018;ESP18-0071

[4] Kanjilal S, Cho TA, Piantadosi A. Diagnostic testing in central nervous system infection. Seminars in Neurology. 2019;**39**(3):297-311

[5] Sigfrid L, Perfect C, Rojek A, Longuere K-S, Lipworth S, Harriss E, et al. A systematic review of clinical guidelines on the management of acute, community-acquired CNS infections. BMC Medicine. 2019;**17**(1):170

[6] Glaser CA, Gilliam S, Schnurr D, Forghani B, Honarmand S, Khetsuriani N, et al. In search of encephalitis etiologies: Diagnostic challenges in the California encephalitis project, 1998-2000. Clinical Infectious Diseases. 2003;**36**(6):731-742

[7] Granerod J, Ambrose HE, Davies NW, Clewley JP, Walsh AL, Morgan D, et al. Causes of encephalitis and differences in their clinical presentations in England: A multicentre, population-based prospective study. The Lancet Infectious Diseases. 2010;**10**(12):835-844

[8] Venkatesan A, Tunkel AR, Bloch KC, Lauring AS, Sejvar J, Bitnun A, et al. Case definitions, diagnostic algorithms, and priorities in encephalitis: Consensus statement of the international encephalitis consortium. Clinical Infectious Diseases. 2013;**57**(8):1114-1128

[9] McGlacken-Byrne A, McCloskey C, Fisher A, Mullaney P. Lyme neuroborreliosis causing unilateral cerebellitis presenting as horizontal nystagmus in a 7-year-old: An unusual presentation to an ophthalmology service. Journal of AAPOS. 2021;**25**(4):250-252

[10] Paturi B, et al. Lyme- Cerebellar Encephalomyelitis, A case report. ESPID22-Abstracts-Bookpdf. 2022;EP214/#1872 Topic: AS07

[11] Lantos PM, Rumbaugh J, Bockenstedt LK, Falck-Ytter YT, Aguero-Rosenfeld ME, Auwaerter PG, et al. Clinical practice guidelines by the Infectious Diseases Society of America, American Academy of Neurology, and American College of Rheumatology: 2020 guidelines for the prevention, diagnosis, and treatment of Lyme disease. Neurology. 2021;**96**(6):262-273

[12] Li X, Yang L, Li D, Yang X, Wang Z, Chen M, et al. Diagnosis of neurological infections in pediatric patients from cell-free DNA specimens by using metagenomic next-generation sequencing. Microbiology Spectrum. 2023;**11**(1):e0253022

[13] Li ZY, Dang D, Wu H. Next-generation sequencing of cerebrospinal fluid for the diagnosis of unexplained central nervous system infections. Pediatric Neurology. 2021;**115**:10-20

[14] Leber AL, Everhart K, Balada-Llasat JM, Cullison J, Daly J, Holt S, et al. Multicenter evaluation of BioFire

FilmArray meningitis/encephalitis panel for detection of bacteria, viruses, and yeast in cerebrospinal fluid specimens. Journal of Clinical Microbiology. 2016;**54**(9):2251-2261

[15] Schibler M, Eperon G, Kenfak A, Lascano A, Vargas MI, Stahl JP. Diagnostic tools to tackle infectious causes of encephalitis and meningoencephalitis in immunocompetent adults in Europe. Clinical Microbiology and Infection. 2019;**25**(4):408-414

[16] Hudson A, Bobo D, Rueda Prada L, Dumic I, Petcu E, Cardozo M, et al. Mania: An atypical presentation of probable Streptococcus agalactiae meningoencephalitis. IDCases. 2023;**33**:e01817

[17] Morrissey S, Nielsen M, Ryan L, Al Dhanhani H, Meehan M, McDermott S, et al. Group B streptococcal PCR testing in comparison to culture for diagnosis of late onset bacteraemia and meningitis in infants aged 7-90 days: A multi-Centre diagnostic accuracy study. European Journal of Clinical Microbiology & Infectious Diseases. 2017;**36**:1317-1324

[18] WHO. Defeating Meningitis by 2030: A Global Road Map 2020

[19] Paturi B. Late onset HSV encephalitis. Pediatric Critical Care Medicine. 2021;**22**:308. DOI: 10.1097/01.pcc.0000740872.03695.33

[20] Toth C, Harder S, Yager J. Neonatal herpes encephalitis: A case series and review of clinical presentation. The Canadian Journal of Neurological Sciences. 2003;**30**(1):36-40

[21] Obaro S. Updating the diagnosis of bacterial meningitis. The Lancet Infectious Diseases. 2019;**19**(11):1160-1161

[22] Diallo K, Feteh VF, Ibe L, Antonio M, Caugant DA, du Plessis M, et al. Molecular diagnostic assays for the detection of common bacterial meningitis pathogens: A narrative review. eBioMedicine. 2021;**65**:103274

[23] Byrne D, et al. Lyme Cerebellar Encephalomyelitis – A Case Report ESPID22-Abstracts-Bookpdf. 2022;EP214/#1872 Topic: AS07

[24] Paturi B, et al. Sudden And Unexpected Infant Death With Group A Streptococus ESPID abstract book 2018 (Abstract No. ESP18-0569)

[25] Liesman RM, Strasburg AP, Heitman AK, Theel ES, Patel R, Binnicker MJ. Evaluation of a commercial multiplex molecular panel for diagnosis of infectious meningitis and encephalitis. Journal of Clinical Microbiology. 26 Mar 2018;**56**(4):e01927-17. DOI: 10.1128/JCM.01927-17. PMID: 29436421; PMCID: PMC5869843

[26] Nakagawa S, Inoue S, Kryukov K, Yamagishi J, Ohno A, Hayashida K, et al. Rapid sequencing-based diagnosis of infectious bacterial species from meningitis patients in Zambia. Clinical & Translational Immunology. 2019;**8**(11):e01087

[27] Buono SA, Kelly RJ, Topaz N, Retchless AC, Silva H, Chen A, et al. Web-based genome analysis of bacterial meningitis pathogens for public health applications using the bacterial meningitis genomic analysis platform (BMGAP). Frontiers in Genetics. 2020;**11**:601870

[28] Jolley KA, Bray JE, Maiden MCJ. Open-access bacterial population genomics: BIGSdb software, the PubMLST.org website and their applications. Wellcome Open Research. 24 Sep 2018;**3**:124. DOI: 10.12688/wellcomeopenres.14826.1. PMID: 30345391; PMCID: PMC6192448

Chapter 5

Complementary Technologies for CSF Biomarker Analysis

Li Zhang

Abstract

Cerebrospinal fluid (CSF) is a metabolically active body fluid that contains rich categories of circulating biomarkers, including cells (e.g., leukocytes, cancer cells), extracellular vesicles (e.g., apoptotic bodies, microvesicles and exosomes) and molecules (e.g., amyloid β aggregates, tau proteins, microRNAs and interleukins). These biomarkers have been studied in patients with various neurologic diseases such as seizure disorders, Alzheimer's disease, glioblastoma, inflammation, traumatic brain injury, etc. Conventional CSF analysis uses flow cytometry, ELISA, mass spectroscopy qPCR, etc. for biomarker profiling. These approaches can provide comprehensive proteomics or transcriptomics analyses but require large sample volume, bulky and expensive equipment, and extensive processing and/or detection time. With emerging micro/nanotechnologies, new opportunities have been offered for rapid, accurate, and early diagnostics. These new technologies, including microfluidic system, magnetic biosensors (e.g., μNMR, μHall, GMR), optical biosensors (e.g., SPR), and electrochemical biosensors, can provide size-matching methodologies for biomarker isolation and detection in complex bio-fluids.

Keywords: micro/nanotechnologies, *in vitro* diagnostics (IVD), extracellular vesicles (EVs), CSF analysis, Alzheimer's disease

1. Introduction

The cerebrospinal fluid (CSF) is a metabolically active biofluid in direct contact with the extracellular matrix of the brain, which plays a significant role in buffering the physiological and pathological changes of the central nervous system [1]. CSF analysis of multiple biomarkers in CSF, including cells, extracellular vesicles (EVs), and free-floating molecules, could provide an accurate and sensitive approach to reflect possible brain diseases. For example, circulating tumor cells (CTCs) and circulating tumor DNAs in CSF can relate to multiple brain tumors or tumors with brain metastases [2]. Levels of several proteins, including tau protein, γ-Enolase, S100-B, glial fibrillary acidic protein, and neurofilament light polypeptide, can be affected by traumatic brain injury [3]. Elevated leukocyte count and increased oligoclonal IgG bands can be utilized for diagnosis of multiple sclerosis [4]. The ratio of two amyloid β (Aβ) proteins, that is. Aβ42/Aβ40 [5], and the order of Aβ aggregates [6] are related to the progression of Alzheimer's disease (AD).

IntechOpen

However, the heterogeneities of these multi-scale biomarkers in concentration, size molecular components, etc. pose significant challenges for their specific identifications and clinical translations. Conventional biomarker analysis techniques, such as flow cytometry [7], qPCR [8], mass spectroscopy [9, 10], and ELISA, usually mismatch in size, concentration, and/or mode of detection and require large sample volume, bulky equipment, and extensive processing steps, making them limited for fast and accurate clinical *in vitro* diagnostics (IVD). To address such challenges, researchers are exploring size-matching technologies to design complementary assay strategies. These strategies are well-designed to unmask the fine features of circulating biomarkers, as well as to be miniaturized for integrated IVD applications.

In this chapter, we first discuss the biogenesis of the circulating biomarkers in CSF and their correlations to possible brain diseases. Beyond the concentration, multidimensional information, including 3D structure, molecular activity, and association with external environment, can reflect disease pathologies. Then, we introduce typical complementary technologies and assay designs for CSF biomarker detection. Different scales of micro-, nano-, and molecular technologies are included. Finally, we discuss the challenge and outlook of CSF analysis as a routine liquid biopsy for clinical applications.

2. Biogenesis and pathology of CSF biomarkers

CSF not only mechanically protects CNS but also plays significant roles in facilitating its metabolism and communication with the peripheral system. Enormous metabolites and messenger bio-entities were secreted into the systemic circulation. These circulating biomarkers consist entire cells, such as immune cells and CTCs, EVs, and free-floating molecules, such as proteins and nucleic acids. Their biophysical and biomolecular properties can provide a large amount of physiological information to reflect multiple diseases. Here, we discuss about the biogenesis of multi-scale biomarkers in CSF and their disease-reflective properties.

2.1 Circulating tumor cells (CTCs) and immune cells

CTCs, disseminated from primary tumor cells, can reach CSF through hematogenous spread or migration along perineural or perivascular spaces [11]. In circulations, CTCs can exist as single cells or cell clusters, both forms show brain metastatic potential. The CTCs are relatively stiffer than blood cells, larger in size (> 10 μm), and rare in numbers. CTCs carry multiple membrane molecular biomarkers for identifications of different cancers, such as IL-13 for glioma, HER2 for lung cancer, and ovarian cancer [12]. Comprehensive CSF cytology characterizing the quantity, biophysical, and biochemical properties of CTCs can provide clear cancer identifications, progressions, and treatment evaluations.

Immune cells exit blood and enter CSF through meningeal tissue and/or choroid plexus, where the CSF is produced. The immune cells in CSF are extremely few in numbers due to the blood-CSF barrier [13]. Predominated by CD4+ T cells, CSF immune cell subsets comprise CD8+ T cells, B cells, plasmablasts, monocytes NK cells, etc. [14]. The amount/ratio of these cell subpopulations and their fine features can be affected by multiple neurologic diseases, including brain cancers, neuroinflammatory diseases, autoimmune disorders, and neurodegenerative diseases [15].

2.2 Extracellular vesicles (EVs)

EVs include microvesicles (0.2 ~ 2 μm) and exosomes (10 ~ 200 nm) secreted from living cells, and apoptotic bodies released from dying cells. EVs are relatively small and very heterogeneous in molecular compositions. EVs are generated to facilitate intercellular communication; thus, they carry rich constituent biomarkers reflecting original cells and acquired biomarkers upon association with the extracellular microenvironment [16]. These biomarkers deeply correlate to various pathological processes in many diseases, including AD [17], Parkinson's disease (PD) [18], virus infection [19], multiple sclerosis [4], etc.

2.3 Free-floating molecules

In addition to the relatively large cells and EVs, numerous brain-derived molecules are secreted to CSF, including nucleic acids and proteins. These molecules show high heterogeneity in quantity and modifications, which are utilized to reflect multiple physiologies/pathologies. For example, cell-free DNA (cfDNA) analyses of copy number variations, mutations, and methylation can be used to identify tumors with different origins [20], showing higher sensitivity than detecting CTCs and lower backgrounds due to lower levels of normal cfDNA [21]. Abnormal total CSF protein levels can be caused by multiple diseases such as strokes, infections, and CSF leaks [22]. For particular diseases, specific protein biomarkers can demonstrate distinct patterns. For example, tau protein levels and Aβ protein ratio are correlated to the progression of multiple neurodegenerative diseases, such as PD and AD [23].

3. Complementary technologies for CSF biomarker analysis

Circulating CSF biomarkers are very heterogeneous in size, concentration, and molecular expressions. To accommodate such a big spectrum of biological differences, multi-scale complementary isolation/enrichment and specific detection technologies were developed.

3.1 Micro-scale technologies

For micro-scale manipulations, microfluidics technology has been the research focus ascribed to its easy fabrication and high programmability [24]. Such microfluidic devices are normally constructed by direct patterning (e.g., laser cutting) of polymethyl methacrylate (PMMA), polyethylene terephthalate (PET), Teflon, etc., or by mold transferring using polydimethylsiloxane (PDMS) (i.e., soft lithography), where the master molds are prepared using photolithography or 3D printing approaches. Assisted by the fluidic manipulation with these micron devices, CTCs and/or immune cells are isolated and enriched, according to their characteristic biophysical and biochemical properties, from the complex biofluid of CSF. Specifically, the isolation strategies comprise size-based filtration [25], mass-based inertial sorting [26], and affinity-based capturing. For example, Turetsky et al. [27] fabricated a type of butterfly-shape trap with a 4-μm gap to capture individual lymphocytes in CSF, while smaller cells, such as erythrocytes, were allowed to pass through. Specifically, the cells were harvested and trapped on chip without preprocessing. In addition, CTCs are characterized with multiple specific molecular signatures for enrichment and tumor subtyping [28] such as epithelial cell adhesion molecule (EpCAM), membrane-bound mucin (MUC1), and ephrin receptor (EphB4). As reported by Ruan et al. [29], they selected CSF CTCs from background lymphocytes by fluorescently labeling Calcein blue AM (+) and CD45 (−) antigens.

For specific detections, microelectronics and micromechanics systems are constructed using microelectrodes and cantilevers. Shao et al. [30] developed an optimized field-effect transistor (FET) sensor to rapidly diagnose CSF leakage by detecting beta2-transferrin. Compared to conventional gel electrophoresis, such new technology demonstrated higher sensitivity and greatly shortened the detection time. Chae et al. [31] proposed a microslit-embedded cantilever sensor to detect Aβ proteins. Such configuration overcoming a major drawback in liquid environment showed excellent sensing performance as an AD diagnostic tool candidate.

3.2 Nanoscale technologies

For submicron-scale actuations, various nanodevices and nanomaterials were physically fabricated (top-down) [32] or chemically synthesized (bottom-up) [33]. The top-down technologies fabricate sophisticated nanodevices by printing a nanopattern onto a shapable film structure [34]. These technologies include nanoimprint lithography, focused ion beam lithography, electron beam lithography, etc. Through well-designed structural and material configurations, these nanodevices can demonstrate specific near-field effects within several to hundreds of nanometer region (e.g., surface plasmon resonance [35], giant magnetoresistance effect [36], and micro-Hall effect [37]). Taking advantages of such size-complement nano-effects, cell organelles [38], EVs [39], and macromolecules [40] can be identified with high sensitivity. Kavungal et al. [41] developed a nanoplasmonic metasurface biosensor for structural detection of misfolded proteins in CSF. The sensor was integrated into a microfluidic system to enable multiplexed and simultaneous monitoring of multiple pathology-related biomarkers.

The bottom-up technologies constructed nanomaterials with various morphologies, compositions, and ordered crystal structures. These nanomaterials can exhibit tailored optical, electric, and/or magnetic properties and can act as a modular unit in sophisticated assay strategies. Georganopoulou et al. [42] designed a bio-barcode assay involving DNA-modified Au nanoparticles and magnetic microparticles to selectively separate and detect Aβ-derived diffusible ligands in clinical CSF samples. The limit of detection reached ~100 aM, making the assay a promising diagnostic tool for AD.

3.3 Molecule-scale technologies

For direct molecular manipulation, biological nanotechnologies, including DNA origami, molecular switch, and molecular circuitry, are emerging as promising tools [43, 44]. With these technologies, complex biological sensing systems with tailored structural and biochemical characteristics can be engineered through multiple molecular interactions, such as covalent bonds, hydrogen bonds, hydrophobic interactions, and Van der Waals forces. Upon interactions with target biomarker, the molecular sensors can report the molecular event as obvious changes in its optical, electric, and/or chemical properties. Dammer et al. [45] utilized multiple proteomic technologies to discover AD biomarkers in CSF and plasma, showing the promising capacity of cross-platform proteomics for AD biomarker development. Jin et al. [46] and Bruzek et al. [47] applied nanopore sequencing to detect infection and cancer, respectively. High sensitivities were enabled by the nanopore technology for early-stage diagnosis and treatment monitoring.

4. Conclusions

In conclusion, the emerging micro- and nanotechnologies are complementary to the heterogeneous biophysical and biomolecular properties of CSF biomarkers, accelerating the development of IVD for neurological diseases. In this chapter, we briefly concluded the biogenesis and disease relations of CSF biomarkers, that is. tumor and immune cells, EVs, and free-floating molecules. These biomarkers are heterogeneous in size, concentration, and molecular components, requiring well-designed technologies for precise detection. Then, we introduced recent micro-, nano-, and molecular technologies that have been applied for CSF biomarker analysis. Precise target manipulations and specific detections were achieved with these size and property complementary technologies.

In future, there are several directions for CSF biomarker analysis. First, there are multiple commercial kits/technologies for blood biopsy, yet not available for CSF analysis. A fast and fluent transduction could be achieved in considering the compositional and concentration difference between these two types of bio-liquids. Second, the clinical translation of these technologies must fulfill important performance criteria, including analytical validity, clinical validity, and clinical utility [48]. Proof of these properties should be provided in accelerating their incorporation into routine clinical procedures. Finally, the invasiveness of CSF sampling is always hindering the wide applications of CSF analysis, as compared to blood biopsy [49]. A safe and non- or less invasive sampling technique could largely benefit CSF-based IVD applications.

Acknowledgements

This work was supported in part by funding from the National University of Singapore (NUS), NUS Research Scholarship.

Conflict of interest

The authors declare no conflict of interest.

Author details

Li Zhang[1,2*]

1 Institute for Health Innovation and Technology, National University of Singapore, Singapore

2 Department of Biomedical Engineering, National University of Singapore, Singapore

*Address all correspondence to: li.zhang@nus.edu.sg

References

[1] Johanson CE, Duncan JA, Klinge PM, Brinker T, Stopa EG, Silverberg GD. Multiplicity of cerebrospinal fluid functions: New challenges in health and disease. Cerebrospinal Fluid Research. 2008;**5**(1):10. DOI: 10.1186/1743-8454-5-10

[2] van Bussel MTJ et al. Circulating epithelial tumor cell analysis in CSF in patients with leptomeningeal metastases. Neurology. 2020;**94**(5):e521-e528. DOI: 10.1212/WNL.0000000000008751

[3] Zetterberg H, Smith DH, Blennow K. Biomarkers of mild traumatic brain injury in cerebrospinal fluid and blood. Nature Reviews. Neurology. 2013;**9**(4):201-210. DOI: 10.1038/nrneurol.2013.9

[4] Stangel M, Fredrikson S, Meinl E, Petzold A, Stüve O, Tumani H. The utility of cerebrospinal fluid analysis in patients with multiple sclerosis. Nature Reviews. Neurology. 2013;**9**(5):267-276. DOI: 10.1038/nrneurol.2013.41

[5] Wang X, Sun Y, Li T, Cai Y, Han Y. Amyloid-β as a blood biomarker for Alzheimer's disease: A review of recent literature. Journal of Alzheimer's Disease. 2020;**73**(3):819-832. DOI: 10.3233/JAD-190714

[6] Knowles TPJ, Vendruscolo M, Dobson CM. The amyloid state and its association with protein misfolding diseases. Nature Reviews. Molecular Cell Biology. 2014;**15**(6):384-396. DOI: 10.1038/nrm3810

[7] Benoist C, Hacohen N. Flow cytometry, amped up. Science. 2011;**332**(6030):677-678. DOI: 10.1126/science.1206351

[8] Podlesniy P, Trullas R. Biomarkers in cerebrospinal fluid: Analysis of cell-free circulating mitochondrial DNA by digital PCR. Methods in Molecular Biology Clifton NJ. 2018;**1768**:111-126. DOI: 10.1007/978-1-4939-7778-9_7

[9] Begcevic I, Brinc D, Drabovich AP, Batruch I, Diamandis EP. Identification of brain-enriched proteins in the cerebrospinal fluid proteome by LC-MS/MS profiling and mining of the human protein atlas. Clinical Proteomics. 2016;**13**:11. DOI: 10.1186/s12014-016-9111-3

[10] Karayel O et al. Proteome profiling of cerebrospinal fluid reveals biomarker candidates for Parkinson's disease. Cell Reports Medicine. 2022;**3**(6):100661. DOI: 10.1016/j.xcrm.2022.100661

[11] Weston CL, Glantz MJ, Connor JR. Detection of cancer cells in the cerebrospinal fluid: Current methods and future directions. Fluids and Barriers of the CNS. 2011;**8**:14. DOI: 10.1186/2045-8118-8-14

[12] Lin D et al. Circulating tumor cells: Biology and clinical significance. Signal Transduction and Targeted Therapy. 2021;**6**(1):404. DOI: 10.1038/s41392-021-00817-8

[13] Otto F, Harrer C, Pilz G, Wipfler P, Harrer A. Role and relevance of cerebrospinal fluid cells in diagnostics and research: State-of-the-art and underutilized opportunities. Diagnostics. 2021;**12**(1):79. DOI: 10.3390/diagnostics12010079

[14] Kowarik MC et al. Immune cell subtyping in the cerebrospinal fluid of patients with neurological diseases. Journal of Neurology. 2014;**261**(1):130-143. DOI: 10.1007/s00415-013-7145-2

[15] Heming M et al. Immune cell profiling of the cerebrospinal fluid provides pathogenetic insights into inflammatory neuropathies. Frontiers in Immunology. 2019;**10**:515. DOI: 10.3389/fimmu.2019.00515

[16] Buzás EI, Tóth EÁ, Sódar BW, Szabó-Taylor KÉ. Molecular interactions at the surface of extracellular vesicles. Seminars in Immunopathology. 2018;**40**(5):453-464. DOI: 10.1007/s00281-018-0682-0

[17] Lim CZJ, Natalia A, Sundah NR, Shao H. Biomarker Organization in Circulating Extracellular Vesicles: New applications in detecting neurodegenerative diseases. Advanced Biosystems. 2020;**4**(12):1900309. DOI: 10.1002/adbi.201900309

[18] Herman S, Djaldetti R, Mollenhauer B, Offen D. CSF-derived extracellular vesicles from patients with Parkinson's disease induce symptoms and pathology. Brain. 2023;**146**(1):209-224. DOI: 10.1093/brain/awac261

[19] Guha D et al. Cerebrospinal fluid extracellular vesicles and neurofilament light protein as biomarkers of central nervous system injury in HIV-infected patients on antiretroviral therapy. AIDS. 2019;**33**(4):615. DOI: 10.1097/QAD.0000000000002121

[20] Zong S et al. Facile detection of tumor-derived exosomes using magnetic nanobeads and SERS nanoprobes. Analytical Methods. 2016;**8**(25):5001-5008. DOI: 10.1039/c6ay00406g

[21] Mair R, Mouliere F. Cell-free DNA technologies for the analysis of brain cancer. British Journal of Cancer. 2022;**126**(3):371-378. DOI: 10.1038/s41416-021-01594-5

[22] Seehusen DA, Reeves MM, Fomin DA. Cerebrospinal fluid analysis. American Family Physician. 2003;**68**(6):1103-1109

[23] Bjerke M, Engelborghs S. Cerebrospinal fluid biomarkers for early and differential Alzheimer's disease diagnosis. Journal of Alzheimer's Disease. 2018;**62**(3):1199-1209. DOI: 10.3233/JAD-170680

[24] Nge PN, Rogers CI, Woolley AT. Advances in microfluidic materials, functions, integration, and applications. Chemical Reviews. 2013;**113**(4):2550-2583. DOI: 10.1021/cr300337x

[25] Liu Y, Xu H, Li T, Wang W. Microtechnology-enabled filtration-based liquid biopsy: Challenges and practical considerations. Lab on a Chip. 2021;**21**(6):994-1015. DOI: 10.1039/D0LC01101K

[26] Carlo DD. Inertial microfluidics. Lab on a Chip. 2009;**9**(21):3038-3046. DOI: 10.1039/B912547G

[27] Turetsky A et al. On chip analysis of CNS lymphoma in cerebrospinal fluid. Theranostics. 2015;**5**(8):796-804. DOI: 10.7150/thno.11220

[28] Shao H, Chung J, Issadore D. Diagnostic technologies for circulating tumour cells and exosomes. Bioscience Reports. 2016;**36**(1):e00292. DOI: 10.1042/BSR20150180

[29] Ruan H et al. Circulating tumor cell characterization of lung cancer brain metastases in the cerebrospinal fluid through single-cell transcriptome analysis. Clinical and Translational Medicine. 2020;**10**(8):e246. DOI: 10.1002/ctm2.246

[30] Shao W, Shurin GV, He X, Zeng Z, Shurin MR, Star A. Cerebrospinal fluid leak detection with a carbon nanotube-based field-effect transistor biosensing

platform. ACS Applied Materials & Interfaces. 2022;**14**(1):1684-1691. DOI: 10.1021/acsami.1c19120

[31] Chae M-S, Kim J, Yoo YK, Lee JH, Kim TG, Hwang KS. Study of Alzheimer's disease-related biophysical kinetics with a microslit-embedded cantilever sensor in a liquid environment. Sensors. 2017;**17**(8):1819. DOI: 10.3390/s17081819

[32] van Assenbergh P, Meinders E, Geraedts J, Dodou D. Nanostructure and microstructure fabrication: From desired properties to suitable processes. Small. 2018;**14**(20):1703401. DOI: 10.1002/smll.201703401

[33] Yang P, Zheng J, Xu Y, Zhang Q, Jiang L. Colloidal synthesis and applications of Plasmonic metal nanoparticles. Advanced Materials. 2016;**28**(47):10508-10517. DOI: 10.1002/adma.201601739

[34] Zhang L et al. Reproducible plasmonic nanopyramid array of various metals for highly sensitive refractometric and surface-enhanced Raman biosensing. ACS Omega. 2018;**3**(10):14181-14187. DOI: 10.1021/acsomega.7b02016

[35] Mayer KM, Hafner JH. Localized surface plasmon resonance sensors. Chemical Reviews. 2011;**111**(6):3828-3857. DOI: 10.1021/cr100313v

[36] Wang Z et al. Dual-selective magnetic analysis of extracellular vesicle glycans. Matter. 2020;**2**(1):150-166. DOI: 10.1016/j.matt.2019.10.018

[37] Issadore D et al. Ultrasensitive clinical enumeration of rare cells ex vivo using a micro-hall detector. Science Translational Medicine. 2012;**4**(141):141ra92. DOI: 10.1126/scitranslmed.3003747

[38] Zhang L et al. Plasmonic Al nanopyramid array sensor for monitoring the attaching and spreading of cells. Sensors and Actuators B: Chemical. 2019;**279**:503-508. DOI: 10.1016/j.snb.2018.10.023

[39] Chin LK et al. Plasmonic sensors for extracellular vesicle analysis: From scientific development to translational research. ACS Nano. 2020;**14**(11):14528-14548. DOI: 10.1021/acsnano.0c07581

[40] Li W et al. Aluminum nanopyramid array with tunable ultraviolet–visible–infrared wavelength plasmon resonances for rapid detection of carbohydrate antigen 199. Biosensors & Bioelectronics. 2016;**79**:500-507. DOI: 10.1016/j.bios.2015.12.038

[41] Kavungal D, Magalhães P, Kumar ST, Kolla R, Lashuel HA, Altug H. Artificial intelligence–coupled plasmonic infrared sensor for detection of structural protein biomarkers in neurodegenerative diseases. Science Advances. 2023;**9**(28):eadg9644. DOI: 10.1126/sciadv.adg9644

[42] Georganopoulou DG et al. Nanoparticle-based detection in cerebral spinal fluid of a soluble pathogenic biomarker for Alzheimer's disease. Proceedings of the National Academy of Sciences. 2005;**102**(7):2273-2276. DOI: 10.1073/pnas.0409336102

[43] Xia L-Y, Tang Y-N, Zhang J, Dong T-Y, Zhou R-X. Advances in the DNA nanotechnology for the cancer biomarkers analysis: Attributes and applications. Seminars in Cancer Biology. 2022;**86**:1105-1119. DOI: 10.1016/j.semcancer.2021.12.012

[44] Zhu Y et al. DNA nanotechnology in tumor liquid biopsy: Enrichment and determination of circulating biomarkers. Interdisciplinary Medicine. 2023;**2**(1):e20230043. DOI: 10.1002/INMD.20230043

[45] Dammer EB et al. Multi-platform proteomic analysis of Alzheimer's disease cerebrospinal fluid and plasma reveals network biomarkers associated with proteostasis and the matrisome. Alzheimer's Research & Therapy. 2022;**14**(1):174. DOI: 10.1186/s13195-022-01113-5

[46] Jin K et al. Nanopore sequencing of cerebrospinal fluid of three patients with cryptococcal meningitis. European Journal of Medical Research. 2022;**27**(1):1. DOI: 10.1186/s40001-021-00625-4

[47] Bruzek AK et al. Electronic DNA analysis of CSF cell-free tumor DNA to quantify multi-gene molecular response in Pediatric high-grade glioma. Clinical Cancer Research. 2020;**26**(23):6266-6276. DOI: 10.1158/1078-0432.CCR-20-2066

[48] Ayers L, Pink R, Carter DRF, Nieuwland R. Clinical requirements for extracellular vesicle assays. Journal of Extracellular Vesicles. 2019;**8**(1):1593755. DOI: 10.1080/20013078.2019.1593755

[49] Shen DD, Artru AA, Adkison KK. Principles and applicability of CSF sampling for the assessment of CNS drug delivery and pharmacodynamics. Advanced Drug Delivery Reviews. 2004;**56**(12):1825-1857. DOI: 10.1016/j.addr.2004.07.011